Recruiting in Healthcare

Unlocking The Methods and The Magic

Dr. Steve Passmore

2nd Edition

DEDICATION

Dedicated to my lovely wife Carol Ann; she is my soul mate. I have complete trust and love in her with all things. When I dream and plan, it would be natural for most people to doubt and discourage. Carol Ann does not doubt dreams; she encourages and keeps our team on track.

Also dedicated to my son Brandon whose life is an excellent example of how to be a "man". Without a doubt, I admire him. I also know he supports me in my endeavors. He has his own family now and still takes time for our family.

Finally to my mother who believed her children could succeed.

I live for my God, my family, and to those whose life I have touched in a positive way.

I consider life to be an adventure, a challenge, and a quest for knowledge.

CONTENTS

Prelude

The subject of this book is healthcare recruiting. Recruiting is a mix of science, skill, and a little bit of magic. As a group, recruiters are reluctant to share the secrets for their success. This book will unlock many of the secrets of recruiting. I cover a multitude of topics that reveal the science, skill, and even some of the magic in healthcare recruiting.

Staffing in healthcare facilities is an ongoing issue. Owners dream of the day when they have enough staff and the best mix of staff.

My professional career started as a Physical Therapist. I have worked in many levels including a clinical therapist, marketing for facilities, advertising/sales, hiring manager for a rehab company, director of operations, and consulting. Over my successful career, I approached my clinical practice and the later varied management duties using methodical approaches.

I am a "disciplined" Physical Therapist and manager. This "disciplined" approach includes: evaluation of needs, researching various options, preparing a plan, implementing that plan, and finally re-assessment and refining the plan. I used this approach in clinical practice, business growth, and recruiting.

If you are a healthcare provider, you are probably familiar with using these techniques to enhance your clinical results. If you are a clinic owner or recruiter, you may not have considered using these same techniques in recruiting. I encourage you to utilize this book to enhance your recruiting program. You may also want to use this book in conjunction with our in-service course and recruiting tools to enhance your current recruiting program or to build a program from scratch.

Introducing Recruiting For Healthcare Professionals

Recruiting in Healthcare

Busy work days and short staffing are a reality in healthcare. A successful healthcare practice is a business that relies on its personnel, market share, cost containment, technology, and procedures. Practice owners typically use the services of various professionals such as accountants, marketing personnel, and recruiters for their "management toolbox". While the owner relies on expertise of others; he needs to have an understanding of all these expertise areas for maximal benefit and direction.

My History in Recruiting

I have been involved in recruiting for Therapists and Nurses for many years. My first venture into recruiting occurred about 25 years ago. I was employed as a hospital Rehab Director and experienced the pain of short staffing. I was frustrated by the limited understanding of rehab issues from recruiters, administration, and the personnel department. My first attempts at recruiting were clumsy at best with poor results. In 1993, I changed my career path to work in management for large rehab companies. Rehab companies are essentially huge staffing companies and I became an expert in areas of recruiting. We began to develop specialized techniques in recruiting to fill our needs (at one company, we had to hire approx. 35 therapists a month just to keep up with demand).

In 2002, I started my own company that specialized in developing tools for healthcare recruiters and for management of the recruiting program. I hired a team to develop software specifically designed for healthcare recruiting. We developed advanced recruiting methods at affordable pricing. Next we partnered with the largest multi-discipline therapy Internet job board. This gave a wider range of recruiting tools to cover customer needs. We used progressive ideas and we continue to add additional components to improve our "recruiting tools". At Healthy Recruiting Tools, we offer support services for recruiters and managers.

There are two general levels of recruiting which are: executive/physician recruiting and staff/management recruiting. We have geared techniques more toward staff and management positions; instead or executive and physician recruitment. Companies doing executive and physician recruiting tend to use executive staffing firms with their propriety techniques. Staff and mid management is where the daily patient care is done and where most jobs are needed; that is the focus of this book.

Can You and Should You Recruit?

Is recruiting an effort best handled by your facility recruiter? Should the owner make the decisions about who to hire? Do you listen to the staff when they want to add or refuse to add to their team? Does the manager hire someone he knows?

Recruiting is best played as a team sport. When each member of the team is involved, recruiting and hiring goes best. When you play a single sport, expect to find a few rocks along the road.

The recruiter understands various methods and how to interact with candidates. Ownership sets overall direction for the facility staffing and goals. Correct staffing has an impact on obtaining those goals. In addition, ownership approves funding for recruiting efforts, salaries, and benefits. The staff can set a positive or negative tone during onsite interviews. They can panic or support the idea of additional staff and how it might affect their job. The manager is typically involved heavily in the interview meeting and the daily operations of the facility.

The premise is "can you" and "should you" be involved in recruiting. Obviously recruiting is a team sport which requires many people working together; so the team should be involved. The next questions is: can you be involved in the recruiting effort? I believe by using the material in this book, you can train for the recruiting effort. So the answer for the team is yes for both "can you" and "should you" participate in the recruiting effort.

Recruiting is a Sales Program

Recruiting in Your Practice – Who Has the Time

At the end of each day in the clinic, you often go home late or leave projects uncompleted. Perhaps you see opportunities for growth of your practice but have limitations of time and staff. You feel the need to add or replace staff.

You entered the medical field to help others and to gain some personal satisfaction along the way. As you move from a new graduate, "fresh out of academia", to the "old-timer"; you can see how your "ideals" have changed into the new "reality". Medical practice is evolving and you must add or retain skill sets outside of a clinical medical practice.

Some clinics and practitioners may be able to coast and

survive without growth; however, most practitioners realize they need to incorporate selling to enhance their medical practice. Recruiting is often a major part of your overall sales program. Years ago, adding or replacing staff was simpler; you placed a small ad in the newspaper and waited for results. As you may have noticed, we don't live in a simple world today. To score in growth, you have to enhance your product, improve your methods, and then sell…sell…sell.

Disciplined Recruiting

I run recruiting with the same mentality that I ran my clinical business as a physical therapist. The clinical model requires you to evaluate the situation, listen to the patient, set goals, determine a treatment plan using your best tools; then, most importantly, SELL this plan to the patient. As you have probably noted clinically, a weak "selling" of the treatment plan will typically give you limited patient results. Accountability and reassessment is also critical to stay on track and revise the plan.

Effective recruiting is enhanced when you utilize that same clinical model for the recruiting staff, the management team, and the owners. Many professional recruiters will embrace "parts" of this clinical model; but, they begin to fall short when you hold them to accountability and reassessment. Managers, who attempt to recruit, may fall short on such things as creating a solid plan using modern recruiting tools; followed by evaluation of the program methods. Owners may set up recruiting departments but often overlook the critical component of accountability and a continued oversight of the process.

We live in a competitive world where simple methods achieve limited results. If you have faith in your product; sell it with the best methods available. Recruiting is a form of sales. You have to determine your needs and then aggressively find and promote your practice to potential leads. Evaluate your practice before you start recruiting. Look at your strengths, set firm goals, then sell with a plan.

As a manager or owner, you are not expected to be an expert in every aspect of your practice. Use consultants and tools to enhance your vision of a successful practice. You may need to bring in experts for their tools; but, you must still keep a finger on the plan. Advertise and sell with a plan and with insight. If you want mediocre results; then scatter your desires into the wind and hope for results. If you want optimal results, then be aggressive and use "professional grade recruiting tools" that compete in today's modern market. Avoid the tired sales approach; your need to develop a cutting edge recruiting program that meets your needs and budget.

Solutions in Practice

Returning to my original title; you can see that recruiting is a sales program. You have a product that needs to be refined and promoted to the correct audience. The manager and the recruiter must define, believe in, and understand the recruiting product. If you want results, train in sales techniques that are specific to recruiting staff; and use consultants to enhance the results. We have all gone to stores and experienced both good and poor sales persons. Clinicians already start with a sales background since they use those same sales techniques with patients every day. You sell your treatments and results to gain patient cooperation and optimal results. Use that same disciplined initiative in recruiting sales.

Modern recruiting tools include such things as Internet advertising, direct mail, cold calling, social media, etc. Just like your therapy treatments, each tool must be specific and correctly designed; or, they will result in wasted effort and money. Effective recruiting programs do not need to be overly expensive; they need to be professional.

We have designed "professional grade" recruiting tools that you purchase on a "pay as you need" plan. There is no need to reinvent the wheel but you must take an active role in the sales process for best results. Use experts to help but remember; it's your practice, not the recruiters. Use professional tools to build a professional recruiting sales program.

As a final comment, let me propose my "5 B's of Selling": Be Competitive / Be Truthful / Be Professional / Be Proud / and Be Prepared to Close the Deal.

Contrast Recruiting Methods

Defining the Two Recruiting Types

I believe recruiting techniques can be split into 2 broad categories - Passive and Active.

Passive Recruiting

Passive recruiting requires a lower level of interaction from the recruiter/employer. Passive recruiting methods include such things as: Internet job boards, newspaper ads, journal ads, status in community (ex: hospitals are visible healthcare institutions), expertise in community (you are recognized as the leader in the area), social Internet sites (ex: Facebook), and professional newsletters.

Active Recruiting

Active recruiting requires a higher level of ongoing activity by the recruiter/employer. Active recruiting methods include such things as: employee incentive programs, post card mailers, cold calling, in-service programs, student internships, open house (requires a lot of prep work), scholarships, and using outside recruiters.

Examining Primary Recruiting Methods

I love when people ask me the time honored question: "How do I find a therapist or nurse?" They are searching for a simple answer and method to a primary need in their business. The problem is there is NO best method to recruit. It's kind of like trying to catch a greased pig… you can get a grasp onto part of that pig but the target keeps moving. There is a limited resource of quality therapists and nurses. In reality, you are usually stealing from another clinic or hospital to increase your staff. There are many techniques and I have listed some general comments on common recruiting methods.

Passive Recruiting Methods include

Internet Job Board Posting

These job boards are suited to advertise to a national audience. We don't recommend non-healthcare sites such as "Monster.com"; since, posting on those will often create leads from someone with no healthcare qualifications. There are some companies that guarantee your job board placement across dozens of different sites. While multiple job sites may sound great; I believe in posting on a few selected sites is the key need. You should be sure that you market heavily in sites

ialize in the healthcare community. For therapists, we
nd www.JobsTherapy.com , www.PTJobs.com , & the
nal associations (AOTA, APTA, ASHA) for therapists.
There are a multitude of nursing sites but these are not as
dominant.

Newspaper Ad

Newspaper ads work sometimes for nursing; but, they
rarely work for therapists. These are probably best utilized by
hospitals for nursing, or for support staff, in urban areas.

Journal Ad

Effective journal ad campaigns can be very expensive;
since, they require reoccurring ads of larger size. Journal ads
work best if you repeat larger ads for months to build your
brand. Large companies publish often and strong.

Writing Articles

Keeping your name out in the professional community
will build your professional reputation. It's passive recruiting
and can pay off, in time, with people wanting to work for the
experts.

Employee Incentive Programs

It's positive to have your employees recommend co-
workers... assuming they recommend someone you like.

Social Media Sites

Social media is pretty new and lots of people are trying to figure out an affordable approach with recruiting. At this time, I think they are positive for promoting your name for friends of employees. I also believe these sites are useful as a link to show people more about your company and opening. Use QR Codes and other methods to let tech-savvy candidates search off direct mail to find your social media page.

Employee Incentive Programs

If you run a good organization, your employees can be a great resource to their friends. Incentive programs can be tailored to your needs and those of your staff. They can be directly tied to recruiting (such as referral bonus or hiring bonus) and to staff/brand development (such as training and continuing education programs). Tailor and mix the programs; and, advertise these in your recruiting materials.

Active Recruiting Methods Include

Post Card Mailers

Direct mail can be incredible effective when used correctly. Current research points to the effectiveness of direct mail in sales. Results occur when you build an effective message and target your audience. Simply mailing out the entire state may work; but, can be overly expensive. A major strength of post cards is that a person must at least glance at the card, as they make a decision to read further or discard the card. Often, a well-designed card campaign will be forwarded to a friend or held for future use. My post card motto is Right

Message – Right Person – Right Time. Typical success rate is 2-4 leads from a well-designed mailer and 0 leads from a poorly designed one.

Letter Mailers

Letters are similar to post cards but have some unique advantages and some challenges. The advantage with letters is they can include more information than a postcard; plus, they present as more confidential. An inherent problem with letters is that they may be tossed into the trash unopened, or barely read. If you are sending recruiting information to people at their workplace, a letter can provide a confidential method for the information to reach the staff. If you are sending the information to people at home, then keeping the information confidential is not important.

Cold Calling

I know cold calls have a stormy reputation; but, they work. The down side is some of the leads will fall thru since the candidate is taking no active move toward the job search... with cards they are taking an active step toward calling the job employer to submit their interest. Cold Calls rarely work when done by untrained recruiters; it takes a certain personality to know how to sell on the phone. Typically we see 2 leads per 10 hours of calling for out-patient and 3 leads per 10 hours with home health and nursing homes. I would NEVER recommend Ro-Bo Calls and recent federal regulations limit their usage. At our company, we use "rain-makers" to work with recruiters. Rain-makers work the phones to generate active leads; and, these are sent to the customer's recruiter for closure.

Present as an Expert

I often encourage facilities to "position" their clinic as an "expert in the community". One way to do this is by providing in-service programs to their colleagues. It's time consuming to develop professional in-service programs; but, quality therapists want to work with experts.

Open House

Sometimes an open house event works and sometimes it flops. We tend to see better results in the Northeast and somewhat in Florida. In the central states, where therapist density is lower; these events tend to not do as well. You must do a lot of prep work in preparing an open house. Advertise the event and consider giving away door prizes that people would want to receive. Combining the event with an educational session or touring a new department can be helpful. Read the chapter on "Recruiting across Generations" for some helpful ideas. We do huge numbers of these with Nurses all over the country but I think their higher success has to do with higher nurse density and greater variety in jobs. Some customer ideas for open house events - Shrimp Boil (worked) vs. Free Food (nah), IPod Door Prize (worked) vs. Day at the Beauty Spa (nah), and Tour a New Hospital (worked) vs. meet our staff (nah).

Outside Recruiters

Outside recruiting services are expensive but can work. Typically, they will ask for a fee that represents a percentage of the salary offered. You should hold recruiting firms accountable for what they are doing. Expect any firm you

nderstand the discipline and professional
. They are representing you and should know
ask you as a customer and to be able to interact
essionals they are calling. (On a personal note,
‿‿‿pany offers cold call services to recruiting firms. We provide our tools and "rain-maker" services to assist them in locating potential candidates. At Healthy Recruiting Tools, we work on an hourly rate with zero placement fees.)

Email Campaigns

There are two types of email campaigns commonly used. The first is sending info to an "internal list" of people who want to follow your openings. You build this list through such things as former employees, trade shows, and web site opt-ins. Emailing this "internal list" can be effective and low cost. The second type of email campaign is an email blast using "external list" of professionals. Response rate to these is extremely low (see chapter on "Comparing Recruiting Methods"). The rules for creating this second campaign are extensive to meet the CAN-Spam act. With a limited target audience and low response rate, I do NOT recommend you email "external lists"; however, we do recommend you build and utilize your "internal list".

Scholarships

Scholarship programs can be very frustrating. As a former hiring manager, few things upset me as much as when I would interview a therapist, who took scholarship; then the person offered to dump the funding employer if I would match their offer. This shows a lack of character in the employee candidate. Scholarship programs often work better for larger organizations, than for smaller programs (Larger organizations may have ongoing needs; while smaller organizations have intermittent needs.)   Another fundamental problem with scholarship programs is that students rarely know what type practice they will want before they start school; they may want to enter an entirely different type of practice than the one who is paying for their scholarship.

Summary Chart: Pros and Cons of Recruiting Methods

Cold Calling

Pro

-   Tried and true method that generates results
-   Works best in the local market
-   Build a personal relationship with the candidate and answer their Q&A quickly
-   You may receive leads of friends or co-workers who might be interested

Con

-   Phone numbers are becoming harder to find (At our company we use sophisticated techniques that find

numbers the others miss)
- Requires a trained person who can call, use an informative script, and understands active listening

Internet Job Boards

Pro

- Covers national and international market with searches
- Inexpensive for coverage
- Targets web savvy
- Available 24-7 for convenience of job seeker

Con

- Requires someone actively searching for a job
- Some recruiters are using the web to "fish" for candidates with non-specific jobs
- Non healthcare sites will attract non-healthcare candidates (Use a site that is marketed to healthcare such as www.jobstherapy.com and avoid the monster job web sites)
- Many sites do not market to the correct target audience (too general for healthcare)

Trade Journal Ads

Pro

- Covers national market of subscribers
- Large ads repeated frequently can market a brand
- Large well designed ads give professional branding
- People may go back for months to re-check ads

Con

-   Expensive to place large or frequent ads
-   Small inexpensive ads seem attractive but do not work as well
-   Limited room for text and are built more for appearance

Head Hunter Recruiters

Pro

-   Most have resources and ability to network with fellow recruiters to trade leads
-   Recruiters as a group often network with each other to share or sell leads
-   Highly skilled in closure of lead since they are paid for completed leads

Con

-   Many can be expensive since they typically work off a percentage of the offered salary (At our company, Healthy Recruiting Tools, we offer hourly cold call services with no placement fees.)
-   Some may be "shop" an active lead to the highest payer of their fees
-   Accountability of their progress may be poor

Direct Mail

Pro

-   Coverage can expand to a regional market
-   Able to combine the flash of a larger ad while defining

the critical sales points
- Able to put your message in the hands of people who may not be actively searching; but, who would consider a job change
- Candidates may save the card for the future or give to a friend interested in a job change
- Highest saturation rates, you simply reach more people
- Marketing through direct mail has better response rate than email and this is growing (Confirmed by studies from USPS and marketing association studies.)
- People trust mail delivered by post office over email and they spend more time reviewing it

Con

- Requires accurate list to give best delivery (At our company, Healthy Recruiting Tools, we have the best lists in the industry.)
- Poor design leads to a quick trip to the garbage pile
- Mail delivered to work addresses may be discarded by the facility or supervisor

The "Five R'S" of Recruiting

What are the 5 R's

Recruiting for medical practices would be much easier if hiring was as simple as going to the drive-thru window at McDonalds. "Hold the onions and extra pickles" would be my request while the person behind me can easily place his custom order to "hold the mustard". After taking a few bites, discovering an error, I just toss the burger or scrape those onions off the bun.

Recruiting professional staff is never as easy as "placing an order", then choosing from the menu of applicants. Finding that first applicant can be a chore; and, rarely do we have the luxury of multiple applicants. The Secret of Recruiting is to create an atmosphere where your optimal applicant can find you at the right time.

I have worked with many practices to enhance or create a recruiting event. For a single effort, or even with an ongoing program, I attempt to create a mindset based on my "Five R's of Recruiting". These "Five R's" for a recruiting event are: "Right Start", "Right Person", "Right Message", "Right Time", and "Right Product".

#1   Right Start

Recruiting the best staff seldom happens by accident. Successful hiring works best with the "right start". To begin an effective recruiting effort, I like to use a similar process I followed in my clinical career. This "right start" includes an evaluation, followed by goal creation, then developing treatments, and finally a written plan of action and assessment.

The first step is to evaluate your practice for strong and weak points. Evaluate your overall practice and team. For the goals section of the evaluation, create a picture of what type person would complement or enhance your practice and team. For the treatment component, you determine which recruiting methods that you plan to follow. These methods could include cold calls, direct mail, or any item that creates a path of successful recruiting. The plan component of this "right start" is a written plan that is supported and budgeted by management.

Just as would be expected with a clinical; you create an "individualized" process for recruiting, with the expectation to reach as many goals as is realistic. Along the way, you will assess both the applicants and your plan as you strive for optimal results.

#2   Right Person

Each practice is trying to match the perfect staff to the unique needs of their operation. As a negative, the plan is usually hindered by limited supply of candidates in a competitive market. It's amazing; but, great matches can be made when you search with a good game plan.

One advantage of recruiting in the medical field is that clinicians have credentials with standardized training. While this can give a level of technical competency; it obviously can miss the personality, specialized skill sets, and work ethic that might fit your unique practice.

To find the correct person, I build from the clinical evaluation model described previously. You will probably not find a partner who is a perfect match; but, the exercise of evaluating the practice defines a yardstick to judge hiring criteria and recruiting direction. Keep your evaluation handy for the interview process. Carry the list around in your pocket so you can quickly reference your selling points during any phone inquiry or in-person interview. This evaluation list gives you something to reference and focus on during the actual interview process.

Prepare in advance for the interview by keeping a copy of your evaluation and your written plan with you. Some employers like structured interview questions and some prefer the open ended questions. Remember the candidate may be nervous and interview poorly; or they could be an accomplished "boaster" (not necessarily a bad trait with some practices situations... if grounded with truth). Direct you interview around your evaluation points and take notes only after completing the interview. Maintain eye contact and stay engaged during the interview.

#3   Right Message

When shopping, I enjoy listening to the sales person and reading the package advertisements. A strong sales approach can include a smooth presentation, intriguing starting points, truth, professionalism, enthusiasm, truth, knowledge, and a little showmanship for emphasis. You notice I listed truth twice because I believe in all the points but keep truth resting on my shoulder at all times.

I once had an initial phone interview with a hospital administrator that I will never forget. He started our phone conversation with the statement, "I refuse to pay those high salaries that you therapists want." Wow, that was a terrible starting point for an interview; needless to say, I did not take the job. Personally, I have never used salary as a deciding point in a job and was offended with his opening statement. That administrator should have read some of my articles or let someone else do the hiring. While I believe in truth; the presentation and showmanship in recruiting is critical.

Present the facts but use a little spin to create a positive recruiting event. If salary is going to be a weak point; stating salary will be fair and benefits are exceptional might be an option (This sounds like a typical hospital which the administrator from my personal example could have used.). If your existing staff has limited experience; then you may need to highlight your planned training and educational events. Don't hide your weak points but determine a way to enhance them during your advertisements, interviews, and publications. Never assume your candidate has not heard of your weak points. You must address your weak points; and work toward enhancing them when this is feasible.

Presentation is critical. In our recruiting company, one of our tools is to assist the owner or manager with effective advertisement for post card mailers, Internet ads, and cold calls. We offer multiple recruiting tools for practices wanting to hire nurses and therapists. These tools include direct mail, cold calls, Internet job board, recruiting software, consulting, and the best lists of professionals in the industry. Professional tools enhance a recruiting effort to give the "professional grade" results that customers need.

Direct mail can be highly effective in presenting your message to a majority of local candidates in a region near your practice. Design is critical to the card message. You have six seconds to capture attention with direct mail. I you use a post card, the primary sales points and graphics must be clear and address needs of the candidate (not the owner). Remember the six second rule along with showmanship and truth. You can design your own card or use the staff at our company to create a message. Keep your evaluation handy as you create the message.

Cold calling is a tried and true method we recommend in the local recruiting market. Some candidates respond better to a written message (cards or letters) and some better to phone calls. I do not recommend Ro-Bo calls. If you care to offer the best... then take the time to talk in person.

Internet job boards give you a national coverage and can work well when someone is "actively" in search for a job. Use a professional to assist with creating of a message that responds to search results. Using job boards that relate to the particular healthcare workers will generally give you applicants that are licensed in healthcare; instead of someone who is just cruising for a job.

Review each word going out with cold calls, social media, Internet job boards, and interviews.

#4   Right Time

Trying to sell snow shovels in April is typically a poor prospect; but, if you have a freak snow storm, the shovels will fly off your store shelves. I have been recruiting for many years and projecting the optimal time to recruit is a challenge. I can see general trends; but, it's difficult to predict when there will be excess people looking for a job. Two fairly recent national events created a temporary excess of candidates. First, changes in the Medicare payment system during President Clinton's administration caused a mass lay-off. The other event was a crashing economy during President Bush's time, which caused many people who were previously part time or retired to seek full time employment. Both of these events resulted in an oversupply of the market. There are regional events that can create a surplus such as a hospital lay-off or schools producing too many therapists in an area; but, these are typically regional and of a shorter term.

I believe there are some general trends that point toward more optimal times to recruit. If you are searching for temporary or part time employees, the Christmas season can be a good time of the year. If you are planning a mailer, one great time to hit homes is during a family holiday. Holidays are "life change" times when families are typically spending extra time together and discussing their life and job satisfaction. The same holds for any "life change" event (such as end of school year); it can be a good time to contact people by mail or calls. If you hear rumors of an impending lay-off or plant closure, hit the area quickly with job opportunities. If you know of a "life change" or community change event, recruit the area.

Most often your recruiting needs will occur on an unplanned / emergency basis. Anytime you recruit can be effective; however, you may need to be more aggressive during emergency times. We recommend stronger tactics when recruiting in "off times" or when a first attempt does not succeed. With difficult times, try methods such as "branding" your message; or using multiple recruiting methods (calls, cards, Internet, etc.) or repeat mailers (sending identical cards to the same audience every few weeks).   You see "branding" used in weekly grocery store ads or political ads and it is effective.   One key in difficult times is to put your best message to the best audience... multiple ways and times.

Obviously the best time to recruit is when someone is interested in a job. The problem is there is no way to know when that best time will be occurring; so don't sit around waiting for the perfect time. When you delay recruiting; you are leaving potential money and growth on the table.

#5   Right Product

Everyone hides the dirty pans in the dishwasher when visitors drop by the house without notice. The person who takes housekeeping seriously, will clean-up after each meal because it's the best practice. If you have a weak practice; start cleaning up the weak points as an ongoing process; and begin this process before you start recruiting. Quality people go to quality practices.

No practice is perfect. Use the evaluation discussed earlier to write down your strong and weak points; then use this as your "Quality Improvement (QI) Tool". Address those items that are selling points to the candidate you want to attract. I cannot over emphasize this next point: the practice you build and promote to candidates must address those needs that would excite the candidate you want to hire. The owner has selling points that are important to him; however, these points may not be as important to the person you are trying to attract. View your recruiting sales from the perspective of the customer (your potential hire).

Summary of the 5 R's

Recruiting is a process that relies partially on luck; however, you can shift the odds into your favor. Create a recruiting program that attracts the type of candidate you want to hire. Advertise your strong practice points as part of your recruiting event. Be aggressive and professional in recruiting.

In our business, we consult with practices to enhance their recruiting programs. We provide "professional grade" recruiting tools and promote the "Five R's" in our approach. Our goal is to help those best practices grow while making recruiting affordable.

Recruiting Across the Generations: Part 1- Define & Contrast

Many Generations

We live during interesting times. Rapid travel and instant communication have linked our communities. Information overload is the norm in our work and personal life. The American workforce consists of an amazing four generations who grew up under different world events.

Each of the four generations entered the workforce with a different set of work-life values. These different values were influenced by the generation before them and the events in which they grew up. On one hand, many of the starting values of these four different generations have evolved and merged as the world continues to change. On the opposite hand, some of their original values remained as a distinct influence to each generation.

These four generations include the Traditionalist, Baby Boomer, Generation X, and Generation Y. During the 2010 census, the work force was approximately 5% Traditionalist, 38% Baby Boomer, 32% Generation X, and 25% Generation Y. In recruiting, it can be helpful to understand the differences and commonalities between the generations. These can influence your recruiting style, work benefits, and publication materials.

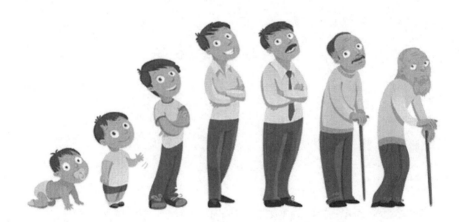

The Generations Defined

Traditionalist

The Traditionalists were born between 1900 and 1945. Their early influences included World War 2, the Korean War, the Great Depression, and the New Deal. Their families were typically predictable with mom staying at home as dad worked for the same company until retirement. A huge percentage of the males served in the military and adopted this "top-down" management style. They were expected to work hard and respect the boss. Their seniority was granted with age. Value was placed on history and traditions; job security was expected. Communication was formal using typed memos and proper grammar. Work and home life were separate; and, after 30 years, you retired with a pension.

This generation still influences our work force in upper management and with lasting policies and procedures. Most of these traditionalists are now retired or working part-time in unrelated jobs, to supplement their income and social life; but, they still influence the current work force.

Baby Boomer

The Baby Boomers were born between 1946 and 1964. Their early influences include the Civil Rights Movement, the Vietnam War, the Sexual Revolution, the Cold War, and the Space Race. Their family life still showed a lot of "stay-at-home" moms. The 50-60 hour work week was a norm for this generation due to their large population and competitive nature. They used work as a tool to establish net worth and identity. They were often afraid to even take a day off for fear of losing their status at work. Team work became strong with influence from the management theories espoused by Japan manufacturing. The boss was respected, as they expected to receive respect from younger employees. Boomers feel rewarded by money and titles. These titles and awards are often displayed on their office walls for all to see.

While the Boomers are approaching retirement age; many will remain in the workforce as long as possible. Since they spent money freely and their savings were destroyed by the recessions; retirement will be tough financially. Also their job defines them; so retirement will be a tough mental choice.

Generation X

The Generation X's were born between 1965 and 1980. Their census numbers were smaller than the Boomers. They entered a world where companies, sports, and the government were losing respect and trust. Childhood experiences included companies moving off-shore and efficiency standards, which resulted in layoffs for their parents. The massive Information Age began during this generation with rapid information available to anyone with a computer or TV. There is little doubt that they are skeptical of authority and the establishment. With their self-preservation mode highlighted, they became more career oriented, instead of job oriented. This workforce expected a good salary; and, don't see the need to start at the bottom and work up the career ladder. Changing jobs to further their career was accepted; even if they had just started a new job or had received some valuable job training. This generation works hard and is efficient; but, may not be as willing to stay overtime. They saw their Boomer parents define their self through jobs and Generation X wanted a life after work. They were the original latch-key kids and learned to take care of themselves. Generation X believed in working to live; not living to work. They are not afraid to discuss and compare their job salaries and perks with fellow workers.

This generation is currently at the apex of their employed job and life stress. They have a mortgage, kids in college, and yet they still manage to keep a balance between work and life. They expect to move up in the company; while planning a future change in career for fulfillment. If you believe it is difficult to understand the desires of this generation, just ask them; they will often tell you what they want to achieve.

Generation Y

Generation Y was born between 1981 and 2000. They have been exposed to news stories of extreme violence and danger during their childhood; and, on the flip side, they have very protective parents. Their major influences were the 9-11 attacks, terrorist wars, highly reported school shootings, and a strict code of legal intolerance. Their parents were often divorced; however, they provided a highly structured childhood. Every child received a trophy for sports participation and they grew up in a world of tolerance for other races and groups. They know the stories of young entrepreneurs who make fabulous fortunes. Many of this generation had structured home and work responsibilities and may be earning an income at a young age. Their parents have kept them actively involved in discussions on family decisions. They enjoy activities which are technical or extreme fun.

This generation has the idealism of the 60's and the workplace problems of Gen X. They have little fear of expressing their opinion and may not realize they lack the experience and "working" knowledge in the workplace. You can almost see their stance...Why show doubts when information is instantly available from computer searches. On the job, they may feel they are working with the boss, not for them.

Contrasting Generations

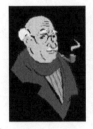 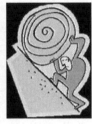 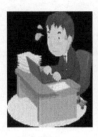 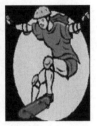

Quick Overview

The Traditionalists are small in the total workforce number due to their age. We are seeing some remain in their jobs, returned into a consulting position, or just entering some type of new job such as the store "greeter". Years ago, the retired were penalized in the social security program for work; but, those regulations have been relaxed so that they can earn additional income without penalty. The economy has brought many retires back to work; as it will also delay the next generation from retiring. The workers who remain are described as working to still show they have value and deserve respect.

The Baby Boomers were born into competition. They were huge in population numbers; and, they learned to compete from their parents and peers. They felt a necessity of moving upward in the work force. Some are retiring; while many are planning to work as long as is possible. Work defines their life. Retirement funds are often limited due to their social climbing lifestyle, compounded by several crashes in the stock market. Watch a crowd of Boomers at a social event and they will be asking each other what they do for a living. You could sum up the Boomers with one word...competitive.

Generation X grew up in a world where their parents were going through record rate of divorce and long hours of work. These were the original "latch-key" kids who learned to survive and take care of themselves at home. Many watched their parents get laid off from a company when jobs were downsized or shipped off-shore; there is little doubt they have less belief in company stability. Still they survived and they expect a good job; plus balance in their personal life that was missing with their parent's life. You can summarize them as working smart, efficient, and with limited trust of the company.

The Generation Y's are newer to the work force. They grew up working or in a structured childhood of family and activities. Multi-tasking is natural with their communication, entertainment, and work. One job is not considered a challenge and they may be asking to move up, laterally, or in different directions. Work life balance is critical and they want work to be fun. If the job is not fun, they have no problem with job hopping to the next great adventure. Communication is fast and they want to be challenged. The future work force needs to adjust to this generation. It would be easy to describe this generation as extreme and multi-tasking. They are the precursor to the upcoming generation, Generation Z.

Contrast by Examples

Sitting in the restaurant you may observe four distinct groups. The Traditionalist is over-heard to say, "Hey Joe, how's the wife and kids doing?" They typically divide work from social events. The Baby Boomers will be comparing jobs and asking how work projects are going; as they try to impress each other. Boomers tend to define themselves by their job. Gen X's are discussing social time and where the kids and family can go to enjoy the beach. The Generation Y's are "all over the map", as they have the TV going (changing stations before the end of the show), while listening to music, and texting to people (some are sitting across the table from them).

In the job world, the Traditionalist believes you should stay in a job for many years to support the company mission. The Boomers keep a close eye on the job ladder so they can slowly climb to the top. They plan to assume a higher job title with more awards and certificates on their office wall. The Gen X are into technology and do not want to be micro-managed. They enjoy training to enhance their career; which easily could be transferred to the next company. The Generation Y's are busy multi-tasking and expect to be given a career to challenge their skills. They are confident beyond their years; and, they plan to add value to the company.

Give the groups a project at work such as planning a "meet and greet" event and you can enjoy the different approaches. The Traditionalists will want to meet and determine what was done in the past. Formal menus and invitations will be created and people will be assigned to give motivational speeches at the dinner. The Boomers will meet and set up committees. More senior members will head each committee and a time frame for reporting in 3 days; with follow up reports for the next meeting. Finally a plan of action will be created with a place for the committee chairman to sign off on. The Gen X's will want banter a few ideas around and want to create a quick but comprehensive plan of action. Follow up meetings will be brief. They will also want to know if people will be paid to attend the social event. The Gen Y's will hire a catering company without approval for expenses. A big concern will be who will be bringing the Frisbee and other games. They will set up activities for old and young since they are considerate and respectful of different age groups. They enjoy their own groups as well as older age groups; but, they plan to have fun.

The US Army: A Study in Hiring Generations

The US Army has been actively involved in creating advertising messages [1] for the different generations. They have recruiting quotas that have varied through the draft, patriotic wars, unpopular wars, and the all-volunteer army. Over the years, we can see several changes in their slogans and posters [2] relating to the generations.

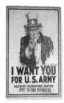 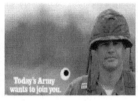 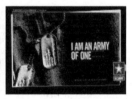

Uncle Sam Poster and Slogan saying *"I Want You"* with the grand old man pointing at you; while wearing red, white, and blue.

- Created by James Montgomery Flagg in 1917
- Heavy use in WW1 and continued into WW2 (Traditionalist recruiting)
- Reinforced loyalty and patriotic idealism

"Today's Army Wants to Join You"

- Created in 1971 (Baby Boomer recruiting)

- Started toward end of the draft after the unpopular war in Vietnam War
- Relaxed new attitude to encourage employment, more so than duty
- Ads reinforced the Army as a job where Boomers could showcase their career and receive excellent benefits.

"Join the People Who've Joined the Army" & then *"This is the Army"*

- Created in 1973 & 1978 (Baby Boomer recruiting)
- The draft ended and the Army needed to promote military service as a job.
- Just a modification of the previous slogans as times evolved

"Be All You Can Be"

- Created in 1981 (Generation X recruiting)
- Highly popular jingle, judged second best in 20th Century by Advertising Age magazine.
- Created for Gen X who needed to make move up quickly and get out of the shadow of the Boomers

"An Army of One" & *"The Power of One"*

- Created in 2001 (Generation Y recruiting)
- Went along with plenty of supporting ads for "GoArmy.Com" as seen on race cars, rodeo events, magazine ads, etc.
- High tech and also presenting message to people who are very confident in their abilities.
- Ads on TV emphasize talking with parents about a career

You can see how each campaign was designed for a generation. Would a Traditionalist be recruited by "An Army of One"? The answer is no; they were into military command structure and loyalty. Would a Generation X be attracted to "Today's Army Wants to Join You"? The answer is again no; they were trying to establish themselves separate from a controlling Boomer and Traditionalist workforce. The campaigns were well thought out and successful for the generation they wanted to attract. The Army re-vamped their slogans and their internal operations to meet each recruiting generation.

Don't Forget We Are Also Merging the Generations

It's convenient; to think we have four distinct groups living in well contained boxes. [3] Before you jump to that conclusion; realize the generations have also been merging and evolving in some areas. While we can respect and see trends for each generation, we can also see how they are updating with the times. Granny may still have most of her original values and influences; but, she now spends hours each day on the computer, sending out emails and forwarding anything she reads to everyone who has an email. The Generation Y may gather news from the web; but, realize many of those articles were written by traditional news organizations, with the values of a newspaper or evening news. The Boomers have observed the Gen X's and Gen Y's ask for perks; and the Boomers learned they could also ask for some special perks.

The Gen X company loyalty was influenced by observing their parents being laid off to job off-shoring and efficiency wars; but the Boomers were affected by these events since they were the ones actually trying to hold a job during these times. They were trying to provide for their families as the laid off bread-winner. Many generations lost respect for company loyalty during job off-shoring and efficiency wars.

Every generation seeks flexibility in work; however, they may seek it in different forms with different reasons. The elder employee wants time for family, while the younger may want flexible time for social life; or even to take a few months off to fight world hunger or another social cause. The Gen X and Boomers need time to do personal errands and may also be taking care of their parents at home.

Two of the top values of the four generations include family and love. The top three reasons for happiness in the workplace for every generation are feeling valued, recognition and appreciation, and a supportive environment. The generations will define these values differently but the principal overall value remains the same.

We continue to see clear differences in the generations but must also realize they are not living in a closed community and each generation is evolving.

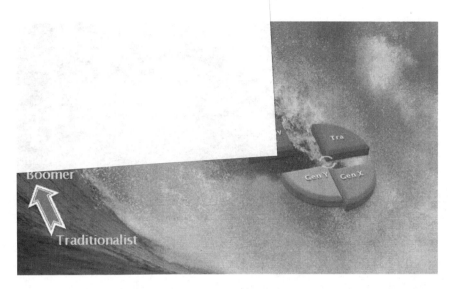

Dr. Steve Passmore

Summary Chart – Generations Part 1

Key – Traditionalist (T), Baby Boomer (B), Generation X (X), Generation Y (Y)

Age [4]

- T = Born between 1900-1945, Age in 2014 is 69-114
- B = Born between 1946-1964, Age in 2014 is 50-68
- X = Born between 1965-1980, Age in 2014 is 34-49
- Y = Born between 1981-2000, Age in 2014 is 14-33

Names [4]

- T = Also called Veterans, The Forgotten Generation, or Radio Babies
- B = Also called Me Generation or Boomers

- X = Also called Gen X or Gen Xers
- Y = Also called Millennial or Echo Boomers

How Many [5]

- T = Census 40.3 million with 7.7 million working
- B = Census 81.5 million with 59.9 million working
- X = Census 61.0 million with 49.4 million working
- Y = Census 85.4 million with 31.9 million working

Major Influences in Their Culture [4]

- T = High percentage served in military with military chain of command, GI Bill gives college   possibility, Expect others to honor their commitments
- B = Started the 60 hour work week, Large population and very competitive in work and career ladder
- X = Parents Lay Off from Jobs, 24 hour news channels, Internet started, Decline of American economy, Sports and political scandals, Internet a part of daily life
- Y = Internet and techno is a major part of their life, Global markets, Information available quickly, Slow to leave parent's home, Twitter, Often discuss major decisions w/ parents

Major Influences during Their Childhood [4]

- T = Very little money in household
- B = Explosion in number of TV sets, Large population competitive in sports and school
- X = Latch-key kids as parents worked, Grew up learning to take care of themselves
- Y = Everyone receives a trophy in competition sports, Children of merged families, Parents structured their daily lives, Attached to their gadgets and parents, Extreme Fun in TV shows and activities

Major Influences in Their History (4)

- T = WW2, Korean War, New Deal, Parents survived the Great Depression
- B = Civil Rights movement, Cold War, Sexual Revolution, Vietnam War Protests, Kent State shootings, Oil embargo
- X = Watergate, Company mergers, Stock Market Crash, Information Age started
- Y = 9/11, Terrorist attacks, School Shootings

Communicate (4)

- T = Memo, Policy Manual, Inspiring speeches
- B = Talk in person, Business meetings, Use proper sentence structure
- X = Email, Web sites, Short sentences
- Y = Email, Text, Twitter

Motivate (4) (6)

- T = Value history and tradition, Enjoy motivational message,
- B = Place degrees and awards on the wall, Title important as their identity
- X = Ask for their input, Paths for early retirement or career change, Cutting edge tools, No micro management
- Y = Work with peers, Want to be challenged, Boss is a mentor, Cutting edge tools

Benefits (4) (6)

- T = Flexible schedule in approaching retirement so they can continue to work with time off
- B = Mentoring and coaching opportunities, Post retirement opportunity and pathways, Retirement options

- X = Daycare and convenience for child raising, Time off for reward, Employment stability, Healthcare
- Y = Flex-time, Cutting edge technology, Company supports social causes

Benefits Helping Retention [4] [6]

- T = Flexible Schedule in approaching retirement so they can continue to work with time off
- B = Mentoring and coaching opportunities, Post retirement opportunity and pathways, Retirement options
- X = Daycare and convenience for child raising, Time off for reward, Employment stability, Healthcare
- Y = Flex-time, Cutting edge technology, Company supports social causes

Work Environment [4] [6]

- T = Adhere to the rules, Top down (military) management, Age gives seniority, Salary info kept very private from peers, Expect respect for experience, Never discuss salary and benefits with peers
- B = Workaholic and afraid to take off, Teamwork oriented, Work up the ladder of management, Takes work home, were warned of possible firing if they ever discussed salary with peers
- X = Unimpressed with authority, Do not trust corporations since parents were laid off, Project oriented, Want work to be fun, Will discuss salary/benefits with peers, Expect training so they can move up in career (even if different company), Expect to start near top of pay ladder
- Y = Tolerant of diversity in workplace (races & age groups), Multi-task in work duties, Accepts and seeks out leader to be a mentor, Prefers to work around peers their age, Job hopping is frequent, Work should be socially rewarding and fun, Planning multiple careers (not just jobs) within their

life, Work with management-not for them, Seeks jobs with stability and meaning, Goal oriented

Work Life Balance [6]

- T = Family and job did not mix, Loyal to organization
- B = Raised by a stay-at-home mom, Live to work, If I retire I will be broke
- X = Both parents have worked, Work to live, Clear balance in work and life, Efficient work but leave on-time
- Y = Value lifestyle over upward mobility, Strong relationship with parents, Diversified social group of friends

Career Goals [6]

- T = Build a legacy
- B = Build a stellar career
- X = Build portable career
- Y = Build parallel careers

Flex-ability Keys [3] [6]

- T = Flexible schedules for partial retirement activities
- B = Flexing into retirement, May need flex schedule to take care of parents
- X = Flex time to attend parenting activity with kids and household
- Y = Flex time for social life/fun, Time for self-improvement or social causes

Recruiting [6]

- T = Discuss history, Show how they are still valued, Keep discussion conservative but listen to their needs, Do not

appreciate games, Ask what motivates them, Formal orientation
- B = Retirement options such as 401K, Salary and promotion, Close the deal quick, Healthcare benefits, Ask what motivates them, Formal orientation
- X = Portable retirement plans, Lots of training opportunities, Healthcare benefits, Close the deal quick, Stability of company, Ask what motivates them, Orient with short sessions
- Y = Lots of training opportunities, Close the deal quick, Offer internships for younger to gain interest, Show different career options, Include peers in recruiting events, Ask what motivates them, Orient with experienced mentor

Company Website Options (6)

- T = Tradition & History, Show pictures of older workers adding value to the company
- B = Benefits, Career paths, Online job posting
- X = Lots of web content with media-blogs-etc., Career paths, Highlight opportunity for career advancement, Show if you support community or charity events
- Y = Lots of web content with media-blogs-etc., Pictures showing diversity of staff, If you support community or charity events then highlight it on the website

Recruiting Across the Generations: Part 2 – Recruiting Plan

Using the Information

In the previous section, I contrasted and compared the four generations. Part 2 takes this information and brings it into a practical level to assist your recruiting program.

Hiring: Create a Recruiting Plan

Most companies have ongoing recruiting issues or a few critical needs. What can you do to set up a recruiting program? There are four general steps in a recruiting and each can be influenced by generational issues.

#1   Evaluate Your Needs

Do you need to add staff? Are you committed to the Process? Do you know what traits you would like to have in your new employee? Sounds like silly questions coming from a person who runs a recruiting company; but, I encourage employers to determine their need before actually recruiting. Owners and managers need to evaluate, manage, and commit to the hiring process.

After you determine your needs and commit to the process, you should evaluate the type of employee that would enhance your operation. While many positions can be filled by any generation; your needs may cause you to lean more toward a certain generation. If you are seeking an experienced manager, you would probably want to target an older generation with your methods and benefits. If you want to increase diversity of your current team; you may want to focus toward an age group to create that diversity.

As I have discussed in other chapters, there is rarely a perfect employee. You determine your key needs and search for a candidate who meets most of those needs.

#2   Evaluate Current Resources

You company has resources that will be presented to the potential employee. These may include your web site, company blog or Facebook page, brochures, office/clinic appearance, attitude of current staff, direct mail information, employment forms, work schedules, benefits, office tools, workstations, anything the potential employee would use to evaluate you and your company. Companies typically should not set all their resource materials to attract a single generation. You have to structure your resources to appeal to different generations you are recruiting, create a menu of key selling points for the people so you can vary these for candidates, and keep everything truthful. Don't promote qualities you don't have. Strongly promote those qualities you possess. (Go to the chapter "Recruiting is Sales" for greater detail on this). Think about each generation and how they are looking for different things; some items are consistent between generations and others vary. Be prepared to market those sales points during an interview and with your recruiting materials.

The question you may be asking is "How can I have a mailer or website that appeals to all generations?" Obviously having four sets of materials would be helpful but this is probably cost prohibitive. Companies like the US Army are able to do a single generational technique somewhat, due to their unique recruiting needs. Most companies are "Recruiting Across the Generations" and need to address all generations.

Companies can address multi-generations by following either a "single approach" or a "multi approach" with their resources. With the "single approach", you determine your "most likely" target generation and build your resources for that specific target (Similar to the Army Recruiting example). With the "multi approach", you create resources that appeal to all generations, several resources to target different audiences, or most likely a combination of both.

There are some key needs that translate to all generations (such as flexibility of schedules and an ethical workplace). The top three reasons for happiness in the workplace include feeling valued, recognition and appreciation, and supportive environment. These shared key points and workplace reasons may vary when actually defined but you can still use them as recruiting bullet points.

Examples of Using Resources

Some resources can be designed to include features that appeal to all generations. As an example, look at your recruiting web page; these pages could attract traditionalists with history and tradition being included. Adding pictures of older people, showing value to younger generations, would attract Traditionalists and Generation Y. The Boomers want to see information on career ladders, reporting relationships and benefits. Gen X and Gen Y want to see a lot of media and ways for them to interact with the web site menus. Everyone wants to see examples of flexibility in schedules as it might relate to their generational needs. Flexibility in benefits could include childcare, retirement, flex days, job training, etc. Look at your company and see what is possible and currently available.

Direct Mail can go out with a message that would attract people to explore for information. This is actually the best use of direct mail to gain an initial interest to explore for more info by calls, visits, open house, web site, or request for specific info. You can also target direct mail during special times to reach individual groups, such as conducting a campaign at end of the school year when parents might be ready to move. The card's power is to direct people to your other resources; and, these resources should be structured to target the different generations.

Cold calling campaigns can provide enough "teaser" information to attract interest. The phone sales person must be skilled to listen to the potential candidate and determine their needs (I do not recommend Ro-Bo calls since they miss the skilled listening-interaction component necessary for success.)   Use this "active listening" during cold calling; interact with the candidate and then determine if the company can meet their specific and generational needs. We use professional phone sales persons who know this skill set. We teach our recruiters to develop active listening, keep smiling, have genuine interest, and keep it honest.

#3   Connect Your Recruiting Tools

You have a position to fill. You have gone thru the exercise of evaluating your business, determining your needs, and reviewing your recruiting advertising tools. Don't miss the next step; your recruiting materials should address target generations and connect. Do this by having a variety of support tools or approaches that you can vary to meet each candidate's needs.

Connect all your to your recruiting tools using such things as printed web address links, highlighted areas on brochures, or QR codes. Have different handouts available describing items that would attract different generations; link these to your web site or recruiting page. Build and link your library of recruiting materials, create a recruiting email address, and build a web page specifically for recruiting (or use our service such as ours to create your recruiting web page). Can I say it one more time - link everything.

#4   Now You Recruit

After you evaluate your needs and resources; it's time to

create and implement a plan. I have written other chapters on selling and recruiting which would describe this in detail. Our tools are designed for healthcare recruiters and include cold calling, direct mail, card design, list enhancement, Internet job board for therapists, and personal recruiting web pages.

The point to make with "Recruiting Across Generations" is there is no best method to recruit a generation. I hope you have seen that it's the message that is the key to recruiting. Never assume that older people do not go to the web or that younger generations do not read direct mail. You can reach each generation with most recruiting methods.

At an open house or when meeting a candidate, have materials available to reference and highlight to each generation. Giving each person the same materials is sure to get them tossed in the trash. Talk to the candidate and personally highlight programs or benefits that might interest that person (yes draw on your pretty recruiting handout). Use the generational information to guide your path; however, listen to the person and you may hear their individual needs. Have people at the recruiting event that can relate to different generations. At an open house, have pictures of different generations working together. Everyone wants to feel they are a value to the team.

My old boss was a fantastic salesperson, I marveled in watching him listen to a client; then repeat what they said back to them. They thought he was a genius; since, he seemed to know each of their hot buttons. He did...because he was an active listener.

Final Thoughts on Generations

We have just taken a long journey to study the working generations. They tend to have different values and some merging values. Using this information, you can enhance your recruiting program by targeting different candidates. Below are some keys to remember in recruiting.

- Evaluate your needs and materials
- Keep management involved
- Create recruiting resources that address the generations (use your vendor's expertise to help)
- Target your audience location (use a vendor who can find the audience you want)
- Distribute & market resources to the correct audience
- Fix your weak points (as possible)
- Boldly promote your selling points
- Connect your recruiting tools
- Active listening to each candidate
- Explore professional recruiting tools
- Sell, Sell, Sell
- AND Tell the Truth

Our company can assist you with many of the recruiting tools. We offer recruiting tools specifically designed for healthcare recruiters. We specialize in healthcare workers (therapists and nurses). We are also available to provide seminars on healthcare recruiting to state association meetings, company managers, and recruiting teams.

Technical Primer on Direct Mail

What is Direct Mail

You have heard about direct mail and wonder; "What the heck everyone is talking about"? Direct mail in recruiting refers to sending flyers, cards, packages, letters, or flats through traditional U.S. Post Office mail (also known as "snail mail", instead of email). Mailing is typically in bulk using discounted postage.

In recruiting, we use direct mail to advertise an opening, advertise the clinic to bring brand recognition (such as sending out a brochure about an educational course offering), and to advertise specialty events such as an open house/job fair. In recruiting we are most often concerned with discount postage, accurate target audience, and effective design of the message.

Mail is frequently used for first contact to a larger audience, personal response to requests, or multiple branding (repeat mailers) of your recruiting message.

Some predicted the demise of "snail mail" a few years ago; however, as stated by Mark Twain: "The report of my death was an exaggeration." Direct Mail spending increased 2.9% from 2010 to 2011. [7] According to Magna Advertising Group, in that period, businesses spent over $21 billion on direct mail, which represents 12% of all advertising spending. [8] In my recruiting company, our customers are showing a shift toward increased quantity and sophistication with direct mail; as compared to other recruiting methods. Direct mail is a powerful recruiting tool that is best used to drive candidates to your other recruiting tools (web site, recruiter, etc.).

The First Lesson: Let's Get Technical

In this series of chapters, I will address several broad topics on direct mail. This first chapter will include a primer on the technical information that a business owner or recruiter should know about direct mail. Postal requirements and options are complex; and, I suggest you work with a qualified direct mail vendor for maximal savings. I believe your vendor should also understand the unique issues associated with healthcare recruiting, as well as understand how to create effective designs for your message. As a manager, you need to be able to "talk the language" in order to make informed decisions with the card vendor. (BTW, our company has a unique understanding of design, healthcare recruiting, and postal regulations.)

This primer will give you and understanding of the terminology; plus some pros and cons of different items.

Postal Terminology You Should Know

First Class Mail

First class has higher cost postage. Delivery time is relatively quick and is supposed to be within 3 days in the USA. This type mail can qualify for a discount rate with direct mail using bulk quantities starting at 500 pieces. Increased postage occurs with add-ons (such as mailing a CD or irregular shaped letter). Information inside the letter can be personal (contrast with standard mail where you cannot add data that is specific to a single person). Rates in 2014 for Letter full stamp is 49c (1oz). Rates for Discount Automated Bulk Letter mail vary from 38c to 44c (2 oz.). [9]

Standard Class Mail

Standard mail enjoys a significant decrease in postage. Delivery time increases when the piece travels longer distance and is typically quoted as 7-14 days * in USA. This type of postage can be discounted with bulk quantities in letters starting at 200 pieces or 50 pounds. Information cannot be personalized to a specific person (example: You cannot mail out bank statements or personal letters using standard class mail. Even adding a short personal note to a letter could disqualify the entire mail from the discount rate). Standard mail has multiple subtypes including: "For Profit", "Non Profit" **, and "Saturation*** with individual restrictions. Mailing Standard Class has huge advantages in cost savings; but, you need to work with a bulk mailer to understand the uses and restrictions. Weight of each piece is a higher 3.3 oz. before adding cost. Rates for Discount Bulk Letter vary from: Automated "For Profit" – 26c to 30c <even greater discounts

with pre-shipping>, Automated "Non Profit" – 14c to 18c <even greater discounts with pre-shipping>, Automated "Saturation For Profit" – 20c to 30c, and Automated "Saturation Non Profit" – 12c to 22c. [9] You many notice the phrase "Automated" which means the address and mail meet exacting standards (CASS, placement, NCOA, barcodes, and presorting).

The rules for standard mail are exacting and the steps are complicated; however, the dollar savings are huge. Letters can be opened by the post office for inspection to assure they meet the non-personalized info requirement, if a single piece in a mailer fails this, the entire mailer could be disqualified and the entire mailing bumped up to first class mail (example: if you mail 800 letters going to the same 5 digit zip code and 1 letter disqualifies... the postage for the mailer would change from $208.80 to $304.80 if a single piece violates the standard mail rules... ouch!). [9] Know the rules AND work with your direct mailer enjoy savings and avoid the pitfalls.

Drop-Ship Standard *

I mentioned the slower mail delivery time of Standard Class Mail compared to First Class Mail. Direct Mailers can often use drop-ship systems to speed delivery. It can save a week in delivery of standard mail. (Example: Standard Mail shipped from West KY to Ocala FL goes through 5 different post office centers on the route to Florida. With drop-ship we cut that in half; plus, everything is in special priority mail bags to speed thru the system. This method results in saving around a week in the mail delivery time.) It requires sophisticated software but drop-ship can make standard mail almost as fast as first class mail.

For Profit vs Non Profit **

The benefits for non-profit postage are huge if using standard mail. The US Post Office has strict rules on which organizations will qualify for non-profit mail status. Being a non-profit club or business does not guarantee you will qualify for non-profit postage. (Example: the local Kiwanis club would be non-profit on taxes but for profit with postal). You must apply for non-profit postal status with the US Post Office and be assigned a number. Also, just because you have a non-profit status, does not mean you can mail everything at that non-profit rate. (Example: A church sends out a letter to its membership about upcoming events and, at the same time, you advertise about a church trip and ask people to contact the Acme Travel Agency for details (now you have created a personalized sales brochure). You have just advertised in a non-profit mailer; your rate would go from nonprofit standard into first class. Assuming you were mailing 800 pieces to a 5 digit zip the postage would go from $114.40 to $304.80... ouch!). [9]   Know the rules and work with your direct mailer.

Saturation Mail ***

Saturation mail is done to cover every household (or a high percentage of households) in an area. Essentially, you are reviewing the geographical area where you want to mail and then comparing that to the areas covered by a mail carrier. This is a type of Standard mail and typically used by advertisers who want to blanket an area. This really has no place in recruiting but can be useful when you want to advertise your clinic to grow business. We have a separate division called Focused Mailing Services that handles this type of commercial mailing and discount lists. Savings in postage can be huge. To find our division dealing with commercial direct mail advertising, go to www.FocusedMailing.com

Targeted (Focused) Mail

This relates more to advertising commercial mail; it's not used much in recruiting. With Focused Mailing Services, we can create a list and mail to customers who fit your demographics. Want people of a certain age group that live within 20 miles of the clinic and make 50K a year... we can build a list. Almost anything can be found to build a list. Also consider if you want to mail potential referral sources, those lists can be created and mailed.

Presort

Direct mailers (like our company) do part of the Post Office sorting which is called Presort. We tray the cards or letters to save the Post Office several steps in their process and the post office passes along savings to the direct mailer in the way of discount postage. Savings in postage can be substantial when all the qualifications are met (First Class savings could be 5-11c and Standard savings could be 19-34c.). [9] This requires sophisticated software and procedures.

Automation

This is the highest level of address correction and mail design that insures better pricing and delivery.

Barcode

The US Postal Service (USPS) has moved into an intelligent barcode format. This allows scanning by postal OCR equipment and routing to the correct address.

CASS

Typed addresses are placed into standardized format and abbreviations. When an address has been CASS certified, it meets these standards.

DPV

DPV (Delivery Point Validation) is performed by sophisticated postal software that assures the address is valid. It is critical to understand that DPV does not assure that the address will be delivered to the correct person; but, that address is listed in the postal system. Even with this limitation, DPV is very important; since, it finds huge numbers of issues such as typos in the address fields. (We use this to identify 10-20% of clerical errors in lists that are prepared by state licensure boards. We then can use other resources <software and manual> to correct the addresses before they are mailed.) There are several levels of DPV and the highest will generate Zip+4 addresses. Lower levels of DPV may generate a Zip-5 only or no Zip Code. Without a Zip+4 addresses, delivery of a letter is questionable.

NCOA (National Change of Address)

The US Post Office will keep track of people who change their address and submit a "change of address" card. Sophisticated postal software can tie into this huge database and update people to their new address. This is called NCOA 18 month or NCOA 48 month. Many vendors only do the 18 month; while some do the 48 month which is more expensive.

If your initial data is current from the source, the 18 month will work.

Zip + 4

When striving for higher discounts in postage, the direct mailer will want to define the zip code to a Zip +4 level (example: my office is 42071-9860). The Zip + 4 is combined with correct address format, delivery point validation, and barcode to improved automation in the mail stream.

Flexibility

If a mail piece lacks sufficient flexibility to go thru the conveyors in the postal plant (such as one holding a CD/DVD), it will have postage surcharge placed on it for manual sorting.

Aspect

If a mail piece is odd shaped and will not go thru the conveyors in the postal plant (such as a square envelope), it will have a postage surcharge placed on it for manual sorting. (Square cards / envelopes tumble in the conveyor.)

Post Card

This is a small card that qualifies for reduced postage rate if mailed First Class. We do not recommend these in recruiting since the message area is small and the reduced card size simply does not present the clinic as well.

Oversized Post Card

When a card is larger than the small post card, we

typically call these oversized. Typically sizes are 5.5" x 8.5" but the sizes vary.

OCR Address Zone

This is an area on the card that must be kept clear for insertion of the proper address format and barcode information. The Post Office equipment scans this area searching for the delivery information. Care must be used to avoid placing a return address in the area.

Compare Direct Mail to Other Methods

Why Choose Direct Mail

You want to create a direct mail campaign for recruiting and you want your message to be noticed. Design in direct mail is all about creating interest in a receptive audience. Recent marketing statistics give an interesting clarification for the effectiveness of direct mail. The ICOM in 2010 reported that <u>79% of consumers find reading mail more convenient that going online</u>. The USPS did a study in 2010 showing 42% of 25-34 year olds said they read mail immediately and find it useful. In an Adage article, the Direct Marketing Association (DMA) compared response rates for email vs. direct mail (the DMA is the trade association for multiple advertising methods such as print, direct mail, email, and telemarketing). This DMA study found a response rate of 34 out of 1000 for direct mail vs. 1 out of a 1000 for email. They also found, as would be expected, a heavier response rate for in-house (current) customer lists. See the chart below for comparison. [10]

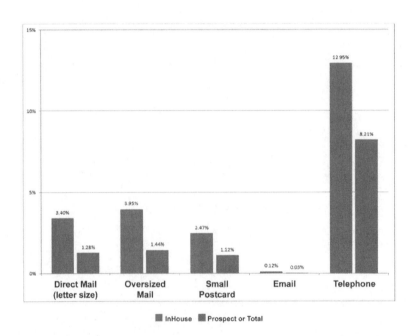

Healthcare recruiting addresses a unique market compared to advertising for product sales; however, you can draw upon a lot of similarities (see chapter "Recruiting is Sales"). Many people in national product sales will be able to effectively utilize web and email campaigns as part of their initial contact due to its low dollar cost per contact, called a Return on Investment (ROI). National advertisers can do this due to the massive audience size in their target area; however, this massive audience size is simply not the case in healthcare recruiting. In a target area (typically a drivable radius from a facility) there may be 10-200 therapists or 5000-6000 nurses as an example. How does that break down to potential valid contacts can vary based on several changing factors? For an example, I will compare recruiting to sale of a product (see sidebar discussion below).

SIDEBAR DISCUSSION: EMAIL VS. DIRECT MAIL – THE MATH

Typical email matching services project a match rate of 10-15% off a set of submitted names with addresses. If you have 5000 nurses in a reasonable drive distance; that would translate to 500-750 valid emails. Sales data from other industries shows a .1% response rate from "unsolicited" emails. For our example of nurses, this would translate to a pitiful response of 1 to the email...and that means 1 response, not 1 taking the job. [10]

With a smaller number of therapists in the area, the response to unsolicited emails becomes worse. If you have 300 therapists in the target area; that quantity would translate into 30-45 valid emails. Since you expect .1% response, your response rate for therapists would be essentially zero. [10]

If we take this the next step to someone in your small delivery quantity wanting a job from an email, you can see why I don't recommend email for a focused campaign. Mass email campaigns are designed for marketing campaigns, not recruiting healthcare workers who live in the target area.

The math improves when you are contacting people who have signed up to be on your in-house list of people who have asked to be on your contacts for jobs. I suggest you build a list of these.

Cold Calls and Direct Mail

If you study the charts of response, your initial response might be to go all out with a program of phone calls instead of direct mail. If you only look at the higher responses to phone calls; you might ask why waste your time on direct mail. You have to look at other factors involved in healthcare recruiting.

First, we have a limited audience. The number of health care workers in a target area is small compared to a general audience for marketing a product. Next you have to factor out that most of those people have a job that they enjoy and have no desire to switch. As your can see, your target audience continues to shrink.

Next, we have limitations of the system. A few years ago, we could find 85% of the phone numbers. Even though we are using increasing sophisticated systems to find people now; that number is still dropping to 55-65% of phone numbers. Add to that the call screening and our chances of talking to a person drops.

Finally, we have a much larger percentage of people we can contact with direct mail. When you factor in that some people respond better to written and some better to verbal, you can see that a balanced recruiting program of calls and cards will increase your chance of success. Cards also have a side benefit of giving the therapist/nurse something to hold in their hands for the future; and to give the company validity.

In the final outcome, your goal is to hire; and, a balanced program of calls and cards will increase your visibility in the market.

Benefits of Direct Mail

Direct mail places your best selling points in front of the target audience you choose. Will Rogers said: "You never get a second chance to make a first impression" [11]; but this is only partially true with direct mail advertising. You need to make a good impression with every mailer; however, the consumers are hit with a barrage of advertisements. If you miss with the first message or it arrives when they are not receptive, you can easily re-invent the message to the target audience with repeat mailers.

The primary goal/benefit of direct mail in recruiting is to gain interest and direct the potential candidate to your other resources (web page, recruiter, handouts). You want to keep your message simple and give a clear call to action.

A secondary benefit of direct mail is to give the potential candidate something to hold in their hands. A card or letter is a message from the company that can be read, re-read, studied, and physically held. This can be a powerful tool compared to phone calls and emails which can be effective but have an inherent trust issue.

A further benefit of direct mail is its ability to cover a wide audience quickly. The message can be timed to hit a large population at about the same time; or in waves to hit manage the size of the audience.

First Contact Mail

For "1st contact mail", I most often recommend cards; instead of letters. It is generally accepted by the mail industry that you have approximately 6 seconds to capture attention as the reader scans a card. You goal is to capture interest; so the reader will take additional time to study your message. Well-designed cards should make the 6 second rule critical for success.

If you decide to use letters inside of envelopes, place an attractive tag line (Header Message) on the envelope to capture the reader's attention. Without the tag line, you stand a higher chance of having the letter tossed in the trash without being opened. This message header on the envelope actually creates a hybrid letter (part letter and part card). You can also add an insert "slick" or colorful insert to the letter to give the person a short advertising summary (key points in your letter, a registration card, etc.).

Second Contact - Repeat Mailers

Consider repeat mailers with any recruiting campaign. You can send the same message several times or change the card. Your goal is to brand the company and your opening. You see this routinely with political ads, the weekly grocery advertisement, television ads, etc. Your goal is two-fold: to build brand recognition and to catch the audience at a receptive moment in time.

Follow-up Mailers

Be prepared with a "follow up piece" for every candidate

expresses interest. There are three general follow up pieces. The first is designed to confirm your interest and intent to continue toward hiring. Another might be a piece to thank the candidate for their response but the opening has been filled or they did not meet the requirements. Finally, you need a piece for acceptance.

When a candidate applies that you have an interest in potentially hiring, you have an excellent opportunity to craft your response. Read the chapter on Recruiting Across Generations to gather some ideas. If the person is requesting specific information; determine if this can be provided. Often you may need additional information; however, don't respond with a simple request for an application. Provide the candidate with information that makes them feel special and wanted. They might be joining your family of employees and this is a great opportunity to start that relationship.

If you don't plan to hire that candidate; show them courtesy for their interest. I remember applying for a job as a college faculty position. The school had a rigorous set of requirements that were mailed to me to complete; after I sent my initial inquiry into the advertised position. I had to fill out extensive data sheets and obtain several reference letters. I waited a few weeks with no response; then, I called the university. I discovered that my request was never considered due to my degree at the time. A simple, quick response could have left me with a positive feeling toward the university, even with the rejection. I had negative feelings about the university from that point. In recruiting, we work with people who talk to other people. Your reputation can be marred by a callous response to potential candidates.

If you progress to the point of hire, firm the details up

with a written offer letter. The interview process can lead to confusion of offer details and a letter can clear up the details.

You should respond to every inquiry... if you are considering hire, beginning the offer process, or rejecting the person. Be prepared and respond quickly to each candidate. If there is an expected delay due to internal hiring and interview procedures; keep the candidate in the loop. Work with your human resources department on these offer and interest materials; and contact Healthy Recruiting Tools for additional information on advertising materials and tools for recruiting.

Direct Mail - Card Elements

Design Process

Card design is both a science and an art. The card (or letter) should capture attention of the potential recruit and lead them to the next recruiting step. Design elements describe the typical different sections of a card or letter. In sales, you should know when and how to use these different design elements to effectively present your recruiting message.

What are the Design Elements

- Headline
- Sub-Headline
- Graphics
- Message Body
- Call-to-Action

- QR Codes
- Logo
- Color Theme
- Branding, Contacts, Required Verbiage
- Cautions

Headline

The headline is the clear, central message of the card. This is presented in a 5-7 words in larger clear font and is the primary sales message or theme of the card. Advertising with cards uses a strong headline, a clear graphic, or both to express the message. Use a font that is easy to read and not hidden in the graphics. When using a letter, the headline may be placed on the envelope as a teaser to attract attention.

Sub-Headline

Sub-headlines use a smaller font and are used to support the primary headline. You will use these in places such as on the front (to balance the card), a repeat of the headline on the card back or as bullet points to highlight primary selling points. These should be short in length and an easy to read font.

Graphics

Cards typically use a strong headline and graphic to present their message quickly. Letters often omit the graphics and place stronger emphasis on headlines and sub-headlines. Study the graphic to be sure it supports your message. Professional photographers and graphic designers understand picture design and contrasts. Also, study your message placement as it combines with the graphic; avoid clutter around text.

Message Body

Letters obviously rely more on the message body while cards focus more on the headline and graphics. With either the card or letter, consider every word and if that word supports and clarifies your department, position, and needs. Each word is critical and don't waste your space and audience attention.

Call-To-Action

Recalling the chapter with the title "Recruiting is Sales"; you never forget to close the sale. A call-to-action is a clear statement that gives the reader a way to respond toward closing the sale. Tell the reader what you want them to do and make this statement easy to locate with off-setting colors or graphics. Let the reader know why they received your card or letter with a call-to-action.

QR Codes

Technology can be a wonderful tool. QR (Quick Response) codes are those square graphics that are increasing showing up on print advertisement and packaging. In recruiting, I believe they can best be utilized to take the candidate to a web site or email link that reinforces the recruiting call-to-action. At our company, we have developed a product where we link the candidate to a web site that specifically advertises their opening (called a Personal Recruiting Page or PRP). I believe you should dedicate a site to recruiting, instead of relying on the company web site, where recruiting is just a link. The QR Code is an easy method to locate that recruiting web site.

Logo

The company logo can be added to the card. If the facility name is not clear in the logo, I add an additional text area with the facility name clearly visible and readable.

Color Theme

Do a Google search and you can find multiple articles on the psychology of color in sales. The psychology of color in sales may not be clearly scientific but is still interesting. Barring scientific studies there are some general trends that you can consider with color. Bold colors can make bold statements, contrasting colors between text and graphics can make reading easier. Also color themes are recognized from their general usage, such as red-white-blue for patriotic or red often associated with sales events from television ads. I will address the psychology of color in a later chapter.

For this discussion on use of color in your card theme, I use some techniques to make the card message easier to read, allow the message to stand out in contrast, or to make a pleasing design. I often start with the logo or primary picture and pick color shades from this to complement or contrast with the card text. As an example, if the logo uses yellow and green; I might use a contrasting background with green text and some yellow graphics to tie things together. Study other people's designs or take the advice of a trusted graphic designer.

Branding, Contacts, Required Verbiage

Certain branding logos or messages may be required by law or by the customer. You can often minimize these. An example is the usage of EOE (for Equal Opportunity Employer). While these are important, the real-estate space on your card is critical and you need to maximize space for the recruiting message.

Contact information is a critical element of the card and should be clear. Give the contact person's name if possible instead of a blank email address. Always double check spelling of the web, phone, and email addresses. Should I repeat that twice; don't mess up the spelling.

Cautions

Work with your direct mailer to avoid small mistakes. Here are a few of the easily overlooked mistakes:

- Allow sufficient space for the address field. If you plan to use automated standards, allow sufficient width for the barcode and clear zones.
- Avoid placement of contact address fields in the Optical Character Recognition (OCR) Scan area. Basically, the post office scans the lower half of the card as it searches for the delivery address. Normally it would choose the address with the barcode that is on the right side of a card; however, if you place a partial address on the left side of the card, the OCR equipment might pick up that address and mail every card to it. (True example: I created a card for my mother-in-law to announce her new address to her friends. We put her new address within the text on the left

side of the card. I then put a delivery address, in a clear white area on the right side of the card. About 10 percent of the cards were delivered to her new address, instead of the intended recipient.)

- Present a professional look to the card. I recommend oversized cards, not the small postcard size. You may save a little on postage and printing with the small cards; but, you lose in professional appearance and space. I have had a few customers require the small 4"x6" cards and none have ever been happy with the results.

- There are new rules for tabbing tri-fold cards. These can require 2-4 tabs and proper paper thickness. The rules are somewhat complicated. Most people are just moving away from tri-folds and using cards or letters in envelopes.

- Card shape, thickness and flexibility can affect postage rates. The postage rules are specific and should be well known by your direct mailer.

- Cards or letters need to be rectangular, not square, to avoid additional postage.

- Small post cards should be at least .007" inches thick, while oversized cards and letters should be at least .009" thick.

- Cards and letters need to have sufficient flexibility to be able to travel thru automated postal conveyor equipment (if you place a CD/DVD inside the envelope, it will require additional postage for manual sorting).

Design Elements in Cards vs. Letters

I tend to vary the design elements for cards as compared to letters.

With oversized cards, you can incorporate every element with effective results. Designers will emphasize either the

Heading or Graphic as the primary theme. With small post cards, you have limited space and typically have to omit some of the elements.

With a letter, your primary element is the Heading and Message. With letters, I display the QR Codes and Call-to-Action on the envelope or a separate insert within the letter. I occasionally recommend a plain envelope when I have to mail quantities of recruiting letters directly to work locations. Employers may omit delivery of mail pieces to their employees if they suspect a recruiting campaign is enclosed. (For many reasons, we always try to deliver recruiting materials to home addresses; only using work addresses as last resort.)

Overall we tend to favor oversized cards but have had success with letters. Each has a place when designed correctly and delivered to the best audience. At our company we offer design, direct mail, cold calling, and the best lists in the industry.

Direct Mail - Create a Design

Introduction of Card Design

I believe the key to direct mail is recruiting with "effective design" to a "targeted list". With direct mail, you are able to gain significant market penetration and thus improved odds of attracting a potential candidate. Direct Mail presents your message to people who might be considering a new job. It's a fantastic opportunity to place your best message in front of a potential candidate... even for a few seconds.

Creative Process

I have developed a method with card design is called "The Creative 13". The process is similar for letters (instead of cards) but would have less emphasis on graphics and more on text. If you have a larger budget, you can add "marketing" studies using test mailers for sample groups and sophisticated eye tracking; however, this is typically not an option with healthcare recruiting.

My "Creative 13" of Card Design

1. Determine Needs
2. List Your Practice Strengths and Weakness
3. List Best Selling Points, From Candidates Point of Reference
4. Create a Theme for Recruiting
5. Match Graphic to Theme (Search for Art Work or Create Your Own)
6. Match Heading to Theme(Choose a Short Statement)
7. Set Color Scheme
8. Create Sub-Headings, Bullet Points, and Text
9. Create a "Call-To-Action"
10. Add Branding, Contact Information, and Support Graphics
11. Revise and Refine (Less is Better)
12. Print a Draft and Ask Opinions of Others. Refine Again
13. Final Proof for Spelling and Errors... Then Go For It

Determine Needs

As with any recruiting program, start with an assessment of your needs. Are you searching for full or part-time? Are you seeking newer graduates or experienced personnel (see my paper on "Recruiting across the Generations")? Are you using an agency to assist with design and mailing (I of course recommend my agency)?

Commit your "needs" to paper to create a written plan of action. Obtain management support of the plan.

List Your Practice Strengths and Weakness

I ask customers to list their strengths and weaknesses when I am preparing an extensive recruiting plan of recruitment. I also review their web sites and any materials they might forward to me. Before you can create a sales/recruiting event, you need to understand your strengths and weakness.

List Best Selling Points

Potential candidates will discover your best selling points; as well as your weaknesses. Maintaining employees requires that you address the weak points; compared to recruiting which is frequently dependent upon the selling points.

Many owners make the mistake of promoting, or working on, specific selling points that make a difference to them. They forget to look at selling points from the frame of reference of the potential candidate. The candidate may not care that you have some special certification (such as JACHO) but would be deeply concerned if your work shifts were inflexible and did not meet their needs (such as a later start to the work day so they may take their child to school). Each candidate will have individual needs and the owner/recruiter needs to have a varied tool chest that can adapt and sell to those needs.

Create a Theme for Recruiting

Do you remember the old television show called "Bewitched"? Each week, Darren came up with an advertising campaign based on a simple theme. His themes were wacky but simple. Sometimes I start with the mentality of Darren when creating a theme for Recruiting. Some of the biggest advertising campaigns have used this same simple approach. "Just Do It" sells shoes; "Have it Your Way" sells hamburgers; and you can never forget "Please Don't Squeeze the Charmin" to sell that unexciting toilet paper. Avoid overused themes and buzz words such as quality.

Study your practice and selling points. If you need to encourage people to relocate to your area; also consider marketing the area lifestyle as a theme. If your practice has unique points that would appeal to candidates, you might want to build your theme around those. If your primary selling point is salary, you might want to include that in your theme but maybe not as the entire message (A message that has a primary emphasis of money will attract people who are only into the money.).

Create a theme for your card or letter, and follow that theme with your primary message.

Match Graphic to Theme

Sometimes I start with a theme; then search for a graphic to meet that theme. Sometimes I do just the opposite and cruise through hundreds of graphics seeking inspiration for a theme.

Before you pull out the camera to photograph a large graphic; I have a few pieces of advice for this. The first piece of advice is to clean the area and look for stray distractions (signage, stray objects, shadows, etc.). Second, take plenty of pictures from different angles since someone will have their eyes closed. Finally you might want to reconsider the idea or hire a professional. Early in our company, we decided to create a card that featured a hand. I must have taken a hundred pictures of my wife's hand to find one that worked. Now I have advanced photo editing software that helps but it can still be a challenge.

If you decide to use a picture from the Internet; I suggest you go to a professional site that offers high quality graphics and usage/royalty permits. There are many sites that offer thousands of photos and graphics (I often use www.dreamstime.com but there are many others.).

Match Heading to Theme

Headings are those bold title words that clarify the theme. In the heading, use a few words that tie together the theme and graphics. Use simple verbiage and clear type to keep the message clear. You only have 6 seconds to capture the reader's attention; use them wisely.

Set Color Theme

When considering the color theme, you could break it into four items: the psychology of color, colors that reinforce a stereotype (such as "earthy colors for nature, red-white-blue for patriotic, etc.), bold colors to emphasize a statement, or colors that tie into the logo.

The psychology of color is complex and the discussion will be expanded in another chapter. The use of stereotype colors is often limited but may enhance certain programs. Bold contrasting colors can make a message stand out (As an example, you might use a black and yellow background with contrasting text colors.). High end graphic software can be used to tie in color pallets to the logo colors. I utilize each of these approaches to provide clarity or to meet the customer's desires.

Create Sub-Heading, Bullet Points, and Text

While the heading, graphics, and themes are designed to capture the reader's attention; the sub-headings, bullet points, and text provide the "meat" of the message.

Sub-headings are smaller headings (often smaller font size) that identify areas on the card. Examples include such statements as "Physical Therapist", "For More Information Call Mike", etc. Use them to clarify your primary headings or give directions.

Bullet points are key to cards and useful in letters. These are short statements of 5-7 words that emphasize your message. With cards; the available space and your reader's attention span are limited. You can give clear, concise explanations with bullet points. We live in a world of excess communication and rely on bullet points (the "Cliffs Notes") to survive.

Cards emphasize bullet points; not text. If you need more space to expound your message; you are ready for a letter. If you use text; use correct grammar, spelling, and punctuation. You are a professional; portray that attitude in your text.

Create "Call-To-Action"

You need a "call-to-action" on every card or letter. This item stands out as a method for the potential candidate to move forward with the hiring process. Tell the candidate how they can move beyond initial interest into the hiring process.

I remember the last time I went to purchase a new refrigerator. Being from a small town, I wanted to support the local stores, if at all possible. I started on my quest by visiting a couple of small local appliance stores to compare products and prices. One store did a great job chatting with me about their products but forgot to close the sale. They left me standing in the store as the salesperson went to chat with the next customer. I left because they forgot to close the sale. They were missing the "call-to-action". Another example is the time I was curious to see if a local facility was hiring. I went to their company web site and found a tab on careers. They made each step stressful for the candidate. I had to register with the web site and give excessive personal information before I was allowed to see if they had openings. I had to work thru these procedures and then wait to see if I would be considered for further contact. This profile process and poor search procedures was anything but a simple "call-to-action".

When you recruit, remember to move the process along and give the candidate a clear mechanism to be hired. Give them a contact person and a mechanism that is easy and clear as they discover your clinic. Leave complicated steps such as resumes and long job applications for secondary steps, not your initial recruiting contact. Don't make the candidate "work" to move forward to the next step of the hiring process.

Add Branding, Contact Information, and Support Graphics

Branding refers to logos, notices, and tag lines (company slogans). These may be required by the company on every advertising piece. In other companies these are utilized to portray the company pride.

Make it easy for each potential candidate to locate your contact information. Give them different options to send in information or request additional information. It seems that service companies have begun to hide their contact information. I spent 15 minutes today trying to figure out a phone number or email on a web site for a company I use. I believe they simply don't want you to contact them. Don't make this mistake with recruiting; make it easy and if possible give them a contact name and information. QR codes are a new method to facilitate contact info or forms. If you use QR codes, have them point to a reply form or simple recruiting page (check out our Personal Recruiting Page (PRP).

Support graphics should support; not detract from the message. Don't add graphics just because you have a blank space. Add graphics when they support your message.

Revise and Refine

After you finish your card design; it's time to sit back and start reducing and clarifying. Simple is better. I tell people that each word and each picture should be reviewed for necessity. Don't waste card space on the un-necessary.

Print Draft and Ask Opinions

You are almost done; it's time to print a draft and look for visual appeal. If you are using pictures, make sure they don't have a faux-pau. Don't print the picture where to house plant is growing out of someone's ear or some garbage is sitting on the counter. Can you read the text or is the font and color scheme hiding your message. Ask others to review the card and see it they have ideas or concerns. Is the message clear? Are the graphics supportive? Can you find the location and contact info? Give everything a quick glance and then an intensive review.

Final Proof for Spelling and Errors...Then Go For It

It's time to print; after you do that final check for errors and spell check. Don't rely on your spell checker to catch everything. I was printing out an advertising letter recently and reviewing the spelling, for the last time, when I discovered a critical error. I had typed the word "all" but somehow replaced the 2 L's with 2 S's. Don't neglect that final check; or you will suffer a red face.

Direct Mail - Mail List

Types of Mail Lists

In direct mail, we are basically working with 3 types of mail lists which are: saturation, targeted, and request mailers. Two of these (targeted and request) are used by recruiting. All three are utilized in advertising for growth; which is hopefully a by-product of recruiting.

Targeted lists are those in which the recruiter does a search by radius or local area to "target" a likely audience for recruiting. We most often use this targeted approach by taking the location of the clinic and searching a database of therapists or nurses in a radius around the building. Other examples of targeted searches are looking at areas covered by home health where we are searching by coverage counties.

Sometimes there are very few people in a rural search area. In those cases, we need to attract candidates from metropolitan areas to physically relocate to the area. To do this we create "themed" cards. This "themed" message emphasizes lifestyle changes (advantages of moving to a rural area). If we are recruiting to a resort area, we would emphasize a vacation lifestyle.

Targeted searches work best when you are searching a local area and not requiring a move. If you have a small audience and a standard position, you need to supplement mailers with a more national approach such as advertising in trade/recruiting magazines or web site job boards.

Request mailers are those which utilize internal mail lists where candidates have asked to be notified of your upcoming openings. Anytime you go to a job fair or student event; keep a listing of people who might want to hear about future openings. Also keep a listing of past employees who might be eligible for rehire. Use a reputable direct mail house to update your list every year and before each mailer. Mail houses use sophisticated techniques to track people as they move.

With older request lists, you have to deal with issues of marriage/divorce name changes which can make tracking moves difficult. There are methods to track last name changes but these services can be expensive. Sending out a small "exploratory" card every year with first class mail, to confirm the person wants to stay on your internal recruiting list, would be a nice option. It markets your clinic or facility to the professional community, keeps interest going, and any cards returned as undeliverable (such as moved with no forwarding), can give you an opportunity to track those people thru current employees who were co-workers and might know of their name or address changes.

If you are doing a large mailer; you should use a reputable direct mailer who can update your list prior to mailing your internal list. Check with the direct mailer to find out if they utilize software (such as NCOA combined with DPV) to minimize undeliverable pieces.

Just a quick note on the third type of mailing list that is not used with recruiting but is used for marketing. This category is called saturation mail. We use it to saturate or cover a postal carrier route; the route that an individual mail man delivers. There are various forms of this method; each having a different postage rate. If you are interested in this for marketing, work with your direct mailer.

Obtaining Mail Lists

There are several resources for obtaining mailing lists. As a direct mailer and list broker, our company maintains the largest database of therapists (physical, occupational, and speech) in the industry. We also have access to discount lists for other healthcare disciplines such as nurses, aides, and many others. We also can create some specialty lists by combining multiple resources.

You can obtain your own lists but be cautious. Raw data lists are full of errors and non-delivery rates can be as high as 25+%. You may think your message is going out; but, it can be full of holes. Many commercial list brokers will purchase raw data and then discard huge quantities of those who are undeliverable; our company attempts to correct the data lists we obtain which means we simply find people the competitors toss out. Some people use association lists; however, please realize these have several drawbacks. The associations only mail to membership which is typically a smaller percentage of the total licensure audience. They also often have a high business address percentage and if you are mailing recruiting mail to the business address; expect some of those to get lost or discarded by the employer. I know this does not sound legal; but, its real life. Employers don't want to distribute recruiting mail to their staff.

At our company, we are a direct mailer, card designer, and discount list broker. Feel free to contact us for services as they might relate to your needs. Depending on your company situation, we could provide mailers or with large companies, we provide list clean up / enhancement.

Enhanced Mail Lists

List enhancement is simply a clean-up procedure of mail / call lists. The procedures can be simple or complex; and the software for performing this is expensive. Enhancement is done for several reasons; with the most important being able to locate people for optimal delivery or phone calls. Another reason to enhance lists is to qualify for reduced postage rates and higher delivery. We also use enhancement to track people as they move about the country (6% of the population moves every year and most forget to notify their state boards or organizations in a timely fashion). With so many people moving, we are tracking people every month as they travel across town, state or nation.

Direct Mail - Design for Success

Psychology of Color

Much has been written about the psychology of color in sales. I believe the psychology of color is a combination of science and of hype.

Color has multiple aspects to consider in marketing for recruiting. The primary aspects typically considered include branding, emotions, and culture. To truly understand color in advertising would be beyond the scope of this chapter; as this is a huge area of specialization within marketing. The psychology of color affecting emotions should be used as a suggestion; not an absolute rule.

Every major company brands their product with colors to

enhance sales and recognition. In designing an advertising piece, you may want to consider the colors associated with large companies and the branding message they are associated with. Red combined with yellow is associated with fast food restaurants (such as McDonald's logo and the interior colors of many fast food establishments). This red/yellow combination might not be advisable for recruiting. Red alone is associated with discounts and sales (such as the Target logo and it is often on TV ads for huge sales events). A dominance of red color might be appropriate if you are advertising discount services but not so much with recruiting. Pink is well represented in women's issues (such as the pink ribbon with Breast Cancer Research Fund and similar female dominated companies). Some pink may be appropriate when you are recruiting for women's health when you want to quickly target female candidates. The primary color combinations of red, blue, and green (used in Toys-R-Us and other pediatric advertising) may be useful in promoting a pediatric recruiting position but not an executive position where a more conservative black, silver, white (as used in logos for Lincoln cars and other luxury products) would be more appropriate. [12] [13]

Marketing specialists may associate emotions with colors. The science is not always clear and may be affected with different personal experiences. Even with these limitations, you may want to look at color and emotions for its broad effect. As a general trend, we would associate the following emotions with a color:

- Yellow – Warmth and clarity – samples include UPS, Subway, Best Buy, and Hertz
- Orange – Confidence and cheerful – samples include Hooters, Harley Davidson, and Amazon

- Red – Bold and youthful – samples include Kellogg's, Coca-Cola, Exxon, and Target
- Purple – Wise and imaginative – samples include Yahoo, Welch's, and Monster.com
- Blue – Strength and dependable – samples include Dell, AT&T, Lowes, Facebook, and IBM
- Green – Health and growth – samples include John Deere, Animal Planet, and British Petroleum
- Gray – Calm and neutral – samples include Mercedes Benz, Honda, Nike, and Puma [12]

Taking emotions a step further, different cultures associate different emotions with colors. If you are recruiting in an area with a strong cultural population, then research color to avoid blunders. Some comparisons in typical recruiting cultures are:

- Blue – In the USA & UK it symbolizes dependable, high quality, trustworthy, and masculine. In Germany it symbolizes warmth and feminine. In Asian it symbolizes cold and evil. In India it symbolizes purity.
- White – In USA & UK it symbolizes happiness and purity. In Asian it symbolizes mourning and death. In India it symbolizes mourning and death.
- Green – In USA & UK it symbolizes envy, good taste, adventure, and happiness. In Asian it symbolizes danger and disease.
- Yellow – In USA & UK it symbolizes warmth, happy, and pure. In Germany it symbolizes envy and jealousy. In Mexico it symbolizes death.

- Red – In USA & UK it symbolizes love, danger, defiance, hostile, strength, excitement, and lust. In German it symbolizes fear, anger, unlucky, and jealousy. In Mexico it symbolizes anger, envy, and jealousy. In India it symbolizes ambition and desire.
- Purple – In USA & UK it symbolizes authority, power, progressive, and inexpensive. In Germany it symbolizes fear, anger, jealousy, and despondency. In Mexico it symbolizes fear, anger, envy, and jealousy.
- Black – In USA & UK it symbolizes fear, anger, envy, powerful, expensive, despondency, and ceremonial. In Germany it symbolizes fear, anger, jealousy, and despondency. In Mexico it symbolizes fear, anger, envy, and jealousy. In India it symbolizes dullness and stupidity. (14)

Call-To-Action

With sales, if you don't close, you lose. You can plan your strategy, execute a plan, and have the best intentions; but, you win with the sale.

When recruiting with direct mail, you need a clear call-to-action. The potential candidate needs to identify the offer and have an effective path to continue in the hiring process or finding additional information on the position. The call-to-action should be a visual standout with bold colors or clearly contrasting colors.

Don't complicate the process by requiring excessive information from the candidate too soon. Finally, the call-to-action should give the employer enough information to quickly start the interview information process.

Eye Tracking

Eye tracking influences placement of items on the card. This is a fascinating science using sophisticated studies to track eye movement and time spent in different areas of the card (or web site). Eye tracking can vary with design elements but tends to follow certain general guidelines.

The images that stand out the most visually, should the images that need action or the primary selling points. Call-to-action images or graphics the sell your opening should draw the reader's attention. [15]

You can influence the direction that reader moves his gaze over your card and where he spends the most time by using graphics. Place a picture of a person facing forward and the reader will spend more attention on the face of the picture. If you take that picture and turn the face so it is staring at an object or graphic and the reader will tend to follow their gaze toward the object. [15]

People tend to read in an "F Pattern". Most start at the left side of the page and read lines moving down and across similar to an "F". They will spend more time on the upper horizontal lines and less as they move downward. If you place a compelling graphic somewhere on the page, the person may still follow the "F Pattern"; but, they will start at the compelling graphic and work down and across. [15] [16]

Time and Quantity

People will spend 3 to 5 seconds with their initial review of the recruiting card. They will then spend longer if they judge a need for continued interest. [16] [17]

Time spent reviewing a card does not change with the amount of verbiage. Rather than creating long sentences; it is advisable to create thoughts or bullet points. Typically contain the number of bullet points to 4 or 5. Adding increased text will just take away the time spent on your most relevant messages. [16] I typically write an advertisement; then start reducing it. Every word or phrase is critical. Reduce verbiage and create strong selling points.

Cold Calling

Keys of Cold Calling

The keys to effective cold calling success are: starting with enhanced lists, using the best methods to locate phone numbers, calling a local radius, preparing before making calls, and using trained personnel as cold callers.

Using enhanced list is a given since you must be able to locate the professional. This may sound easy but it can be a huge issue with the quality of many lists you purchase. Work with an experienced list vendor to create the best lists. Finding phone numbers requires sophisticated software paired with the enhanced lists. If you start with poor lists, the chance of finding phone numbers is also poor.

I feel that cold calling is best done to the local market.

Regional call campaigns or Ro-Bo calls are less effective. Cold calls should be personal with experienced personnel. Prepare for the cold calling campaign using those same selling points mentioned in earlier chapters. Create a written call script with talking points, job information, scripts for leaving phone messages.

Maintain a list of people who do not want to be called or who you do not want to hire. Calling a person who you have dismissed or who has asked not to be contacted is unprofessional and gives the industry a bad mark. Also keep an internal list of people who want to be contacted about future openings you might have or who previously worked for you and had to leave on good terms.

The person doing a cold call campaign needs to have a sales personality. They need active listening skills so that they can hear any hints of interest from the candidate. At our company, we use "rainmakers" instead of recruiters for cold calling. They are active listeners who can present the opening and just chat with people. They refer leads to a recruiter for closing and negotiation.

Effective Cold Calling Hints

What Do I Say

- Develop a sales script so you have a standard dialogue. Don't just read the script but pretend you are actually talking to someone. You can list multiple sales points but be prepared to only concentrate on 3 of these. Too much information can cloud your conversation.
- Practice making "small talk" to co-workers or strangers. You need to learn to start a comfortable conversation,

without sounding like you are teaching, preaching, or selling. I do this by striking up conversations with people in waiting lines, parking lots, anywhere.

- Study the job and anticipate the questions that might be asked by a candidate. Learn common professional terminology that the candidate might use in their conversation.
- Develop active listening skills so you can hear possible openings of interest in a job.
- Be relaxed and comfortable during the call. It may seem odd but I believe people should smile, even when chatting over the phone. This sets a positive attitude that comes through in your conversation.

What is That Name

- When you are calling, it can be difficult to pronounce names. It may also be impossible to even know the gender. I handle this by avoiding the issue. Don't try to pronounce a difficult name and "butcher" it. The person is use to people being unable to pronounce their name and would prefer to give you the correct pronunciation rather than listen to your poor attempt. You will sound more professional and respectful with this technique. If I can read the name, I might start out the conversation with something like: "This is Steve from XYZ clinic, I was wondering if Mary is available to talk". If the name or gender is too difficult, I might side-step the issue by saying: "This is Steve from XYZ clinic, I am calling about an opening we have for a therapist. Would you be the person I need to chat with?" Practice conversations until you have developed an initial introduction line that feels comfortable.
- If you obtain a lead, write the name phonetically for the

manager.

Preparing for the Calls

- Call people who might have an interest. Study your area and determine a reasonable calling distance. The highest chance of success comes in an area where the commute to work is reasonable. If you want to give cold callers a bad name, ask people to drive 90 minutes to work for a PRN job. You are wasting their time and giving your clinic a bad name.
- Work from a script when making calls. Have a starting point and selling points to weave into the conversation.
- Consider presale of the calls by sending out a card to the area. This can perk interest and the cold call can initiate action (or vice versa).

Showing Respect for the Candidate

- Listen for times of distress and offer to call back. Avoid calling on holidays or as they might be preparing to leave for work.
- If the person is not interested, respect their decision. Cold calling in recruiting is not a hard sell technique. You are not trying to get a person to buy a product or sign up for a credit card; you are offering a job opportunity. I once spoke to a recruiter who was frustrated that she had left four phone messages for the person. Leaving 1 message then 1 follow back is the maximum in good taste and successful techniques; beyond that and you border into harassment.
- Maintain a "no call" list. Some people want to express their right to not be called about jobs. While I personally think this is a bad idea (I have been without a job and that is a serious event); you must respect their right.

- Relax into the conversation and give the person plenty of time to chat and ask questions. Also respect their time and don't extend the conversation.

Can You Close

- Don't be afraid to ask the person if they would like to be considered for a position... close the sale. Make it a positive statement such as: "Can I have our manager call you to give more information". Stay positive and smile as your ask for closure. Use your active listening skills to hear possible opportunities or objections.
- Be truthful at all times.

Final Thoughts

- Use someone to make cold calls who is comfortable and experienced in this.
- Recruiters may rely on companies like ours where we offer "rainmaker" services. Rainmakers are great at cold calling and developing leads that can be closed and evaluated by a skilled recruiter or manager.

Web Recruiting

Types

There are several forms of web recruiting that you need to consider. These include Internet job posting sites, your company web page, and a personal web recruiting page (PRP). The advantage of web recruiting is coverage of a national market. Web recruiting can be a part of your recruiting program; however, it should not be the primary method.

The Internet job posting sites are poplar and plentiful. When possible, I recommend you choose one that specializes in healthcare.

Some sites will advertise they list on multiple boards. While this multiple listing is positive; realize many of those extra boards may be small or non-healthcare sites.

If you use "non-healthcare" Internet posting sites, expect to receive applications from non-licensed people. The primary advantage of Internet job posting is nationwide coverage for a low price; but, but you want to reach your best audience. Internet recruiting has pros and cons. A difficult issue with the online sites is they have been heavily utilized by recruiters who are simply "fishing" for candidates for un-named jobs. The other issue is that someone must be actively searching for a job to go to these sites. Both negative issues are addressed by combining other recruiting tools with the Internet job posting and by using sites that are specifically marketed for healthcare workers. Use Internet job site as a supplemental component in your overall recruiting program.

The Internet job posting sites also have a huge positive with cost efficient coverage of a national audience. A second advantage is the sheer quantity of "tech savvy" people who search the Internet daily.

Your company web site should support recruiting. It should present your company's selling points and give a feeling of legitimacy to people researching your jobs. Your web page should be referenced in all advertising to candidates.

The Personal Recruiting Page (PRP) is a product we are developing at our company. While a company web site is important to showcase the company; it is not a good place to direct people to provide the recruiting specifics. Typical company web sites are set to market the company to customers and investors. The sites may include a page about open positions; but, this is a smaller function of the site. In recruiting, we want to quickly target candidates and provide direct information about each job or location. A candidate wants to experience a multi-media recruiting site. The PRP could include such things as pictures of the department, a video from the manager, an easy contact form to request information, clear selling points for the specific job, etc. A company web site can have a section on recruiting and job opportunities but is too clumsy for candidates to search through. The PRP is specific to the needs of recruiting. It should be advertised in your direct mail with QR codes or web addresses. Like other web recruiting tools, the PRP works in conjunction to enhance our other recruiting tools.

The Job Interview

Before Anything Starts

Before you begin the actual interview process, take a quick review of your needs. Remember your clinic strong points and its weak points as you access your staffing needs.

If you have read several of the other chapters on recruiting, you will recognize my statement to review your selling and weak points. I have used these points to set need, promote and advertise the position, and now assist in the interview direction.

To avoid hurt feelings or confusion, I also recommend you talk to your current staff. Existing staff needs to be involved in the hiring process. I am not saying that the staff should interview the candidate; however, they should know about the interview and the interview process. Give your staff expectations for the upcoming new employee and any changes in current staff roles. Be prepared to address concerns such as job security before the new candidate arrives, or actually before the hiring process begins.

Should You Use a Team to Hire?

As hinted earlier, you may wonder if the staff should be involved in the interview process. If you are hiring a new staff person, it may seem logical to involve the staff as a group or individual one-on-one sessions. While there can be arguments made pro and con for using your staff in a recruiting team; they can enhance the process in some situations. If you decide on using current staff in the recruiting team, prepare them in advance.

Hiring teams could be different depending on the organization culture and the position being hired. Typically a CEO level person is interviewed by a team that might consist of Board of Directors (the Board hold a fiduciary position in a company) and a prescreening committee. Supervisors or managers may be interviewed by upper management, human resources, and possibly some involved staff. Staff positions are varied and may be interviewed by human resources, supervisors, and in some organizations by supportive fellow staff.

The key to developing a hiring team is pre-planning. Determine which staff or management personnel would enhance the process. Some people might be involved in simply reviewing and or fact checking resumes, while others might be involved in a question and answer session or social interaction.

Plan the roles in advance and provide any necessary training or oversight. If you want failure, allow and undisciplined approach. If you want success, plan for success and value the team members input. Read our paper on "Hiring across the Generations" to understand how you might also involve different generations with different age candidates.

If you have a human resources director; that person may have resources to train and prepare the team. Use the team wisely to enhance your hiring process; but, keep in mind that you want the process to proceed on a pathway of quick closure if a candidate meets your needs.

Preparing for the Onsite Interview

Review the candidate's resume. Highlight interesting items you want to explore, clarify, or congratulate the candidate on (be prepared to stroke an ego).

Create an agenda for the interview and provide a copy for the candidate. The candidate's copy should have general timelines and events to accomplish. Your copy should set events to accomplish and questions you need to explore. Keep a list of your clinic selling points so you can be sure to weave these into the interview.

Interview Steps

Meet and greet – When you meet the candidate for the first time, take a few minutes for small talk. You have the benefit to prepare in advance if you have seen their resume or discussed with your recruiter. This person may join your clinic; see if you can relate to them as a person.

Give the candidate a written or verbal agenda; so, they will know approximate time table and objects that will be accomplished during the interview. [18] If this timetable will not work for the candidate, determine this quickly so you can re-adjust. Work with your recruiter to clarify time requirements before the on-site interview begins. Be sure to respect the time agenda or you will leave a poor final impression.

Provide a brief overview of your clinic goals and business. (One of the most stressful interviews I ever attended lasted 6 hours as I met with each department in the organization and they asked me questions as to how I would handle situations and enhance training for a software product for therapy clinics. You can imagine my difficulty since I answered questions for 5 hours before they planned to actually show me the software.)

Provide a general tour and include introduction to key personnel. If you have employees of the same general age, culture, life experiences, etc. as the candidate, be sure to introduce them. (See the chapter "recruiting across the generations")

Structure questions in four categories
1. Fact finding questions to identify the candidate's experience beyond items clarified in the resume.
    a. Describe any special training.
    b. Describe exceptional abilities in patient care.
2. Creative thinking questions so the candidate can demonstrate their broader knowledge.
    a. How do you see the changes in healthcare effecting our patient care?
3. Problem solving questions to determine how the candidate would respond to a problem.
    a. How would you handle a patient who consistently

      shows up late for treatment?

    b. Pose a clinical condition and find out how they would treat a patient condition.

4. Behavioral questions so he candidate can describe how they handle situation.

    a. Describe a situation where you felt you added to the improvement of your department

    b. Describe patient conditions where you excel

Ask the candidate what their expectations are in a job. You gain insight into how they might fit into your current situation.

Ask the candidate if there are any problems they foresee that would limit their ability to perform the job

Discuss salary expectations or give your salary and benefit amount. Ask if this is acceptable. (Hint – With positions where salary ranges can vary considerably, ask your recruiter to inquire about salary expectations. You can know up front if this is going to be an issue and be ready to address this during the interview. If the range is $25 per hour and the person is asking for $50, the recruiter can establish a realistic expectation before the candidate enters the final interview.)

Behavioral Questions vs. Traditional Questions

If you study interview techniques, you will run across the subject of behavioral questions. Behavioral questions differ from more traditional questions. With traditional interview questions, you ask questions that have straight forward answers. The behavioral questions center on how a candidate acted in past situations. The behavioral questions are designed to study reactions with the goal to predict future reactions. [19] Traditional questions gather specific information and behavioral questions create a professional / personality profile. Both have a place in your interview process.

Some sample behavioral questions might include:

- Describe a decision you made that was unpopular and how you handled it.
- Have you handled a difficult situation with a co-worker and how was it handled.
- Have you gone above and beyond the call of duty and if so how.
- Give an example of a goal you reached and tell me how you achieved it.

Some sample traditional questions might include:

- Tell me about yourself.
- Why do you want this job?
- What are your strengths and weaknesses?

Additional Points

Watch the person for non-verbal cues. [18] If they seem restless or distracted, maybe someone forgot to give them a break for the comfort station. Maybe they have a question of deep concern and just waiting for a pause to ask. Politely ask or give opportunities to improve the situation.

Some managers take notes and others do not. When I was in my final year of Physical Therapy school, I was given an opportunity to sit in on a committee who interviewed potential candidates for acceptance. During a break, I asked some of the professors how I was doing. One stated that I should maintain eye contact and never take notes.

Do a quick check with all team members after the interview. Listen and respect their input since you asked for it.

If you are hiring someone for clinical expertise, ask them to describe how they might handle certain clinical patients and outcomes. When a team is treating, they must be able to rely on the skills of fellow team members.

When hiring someone from a foreign language or culture, be sure they understand and comprehend typical verbal conversations and written instructions. I once made a critical error in hiring someone who spoke English but did not really understand the language. They hid the fact by agreeing to things I said. This lack of comprehension became dangerous quickly when we discovered they did not really comprehend what patients were saying.

Including lunch in the interview process can be stressful. If you plan lunch, I think it is best to keep the conversation social. If the candidate is interviewing during lunch; it's just a great way to have indigestion without giving a proper chance to respond. Make time for the interview; don't squeeze it into a lunch period where you have distractions.

You should interview in person instead of by phone, if

possible. Phone interviews miss the verbal cues and group social interactions.

To assist with the pre-interview, we have developed a new process where you can have personal recruiting pages (PRP) to highlight pictures, video, etc. of your clinic. Interested people are searching for knowledge before spending their on-sight time. The PRP gives them a guided view similar to what you would expect when viewing real estate online, buying products online, etc. It sets the tone before the candidate arrives for the on-sight.

Concluding the Interview

At the conclusion of the interview, I am ready to make a tentative offer of employment or give a timetable of when the decision will be made. I am working toward closure of the deal from the first contact. If you do not have the authority to hire, work quickly to move the process forward. If you decide not to hire the candidate, call or write to let them know. Be up-front and respectful of people's feelings; they deserve it.

Discussing money and benefits can be a difficult subject. If you do a search on the Internet of salary negotiation with new hire, most of the articles show employees how to negotiate the best salary. When possible, I have the recruiter ask the question, "What are your salary expectations?" before the interview. When the manager decides to make an offer, the first obvious point is to ask if the candidate is interested before you negotiate beyond that point. The next step is to develop a negotiation buy-in from the candidate. Let the candidate know you are interested and would like to hear how they would want to fill your clinic needs. Listen for signs of benefit vs.

schedule vs. salary motivators. Determine what things are key motivators for each person who seeks employment with your department. Some may want the ability to have flexible start times with their children or ageing parent needs. Others may key into research opportunities, enjoy working with certain peer groups, or be seeking advancement opportunities. Listen to their needs and emphasize these items in your offer if it is possible. If salary is the key component, then realize they may be coming to you with excessive school debt or other factors. Negotiate in good faith and listen to their needs. When they quote a salary that seems excessive for the industry, place that quote in context. Their past job may have included travel time or be structured very different from yours. The best situation occurs when a manager listens and has the ability to be competitive and flexible.

Send a written offer or conditional offer to each candidate you hire. Also show the same courtesy to inform each person you reject with a written or verbal rejection.

Summary

This book presents a great deal of information on healthcare recruiting. It provides a frame work to help you set up a recruiting program or to enhance an existing program. Topics covered included basic education on recruiting, insight used to address different generations, mailing, recruiting methods, card design, interviews and a little of the magic.

Recruiting becomes paramount as your operation is growing or attempting to replace staff who are not supporting your clinic goals. When these situations occur, your business suffers with lost business or the increased risk of liability.

Recruiting requires a team effort. With large corporations, this team may include managers, supervisors, a recruiter, cold callers (rainmakers), social media experts, human resources, marketing, and the mail room department. Smaller organizations typically have less frequent needs and must combine multiple duties to each team member or use outside experts.

This book provides information for the various team members who work in the recruiting effort. My company develops tools to assist the recruiting effort and this book explains some of those tools.

I wish you the best in your quest to improve staffing. Please contact me if when you need recruiting tools.

Bibliography

1. Chambers, M and Vergun, B. Army recruiting messages help keep Army rolling along. Army Study Guide. [Online] October 9, 2006. [Cited: April 15, 2014.] http://www.armystudyguide.com/content/news/Top_Military_News/army-recruiting-messages-.shtml.

2. Reproduction Pictures from Multiple Sources on the Web. [Online] [Cited: April 15, 2014.]

3. Tolbize, A. Generational Differences in the Workplace. s.l. : University of Minnesota, 2008.

4. Unknown. Generational Differences Chart. [Online] Unknown. [Cited: April 15, 2014.] www.wmfc.org/uploads/GenerationalDifferencesChart.pdf.

5. US Government. Household Data, Not Seasonally Adjusted: Table A-13: Employment Status of the Civilian Noninstitutional Population by Age, Sex, and Race". [Web] 2011. Bureau of Labor Statistics.

6. Lancaster, L and Stillman, D. When Generations Collide. New York, NY : First Collins Business, 2005, pp. 55-66.

7. USPS. Revenue, Pieces, and Weight Report. s.l. : United States Post Office, 2011.

8. Magna Advertising Group. Magna Global U.S. Media Forcast. October 2011.

9. Postal Office Price List. Domestic Mail Manual. [Online] United States Post Office, 2014. [Cited: November 27, 2014.] http://pe.usps.gov/text/dmm300/notice123.htm.

10. Schiff, Allison. DMA: Direct Mail Response Rates Beat Digital. www.dmnews.com. [Online] Direct Marketing News. [Cited: April 28, 2014.] http://www.dmnews.com/dma-direct-mail-response-rates-beat-digital/article/245780/.

11. Thoughts On the Business of Life. Forbes.com. [Online] [Cited: June 15, 2014.] http://thoughts.forbes.com/thoughts/will-rogers.

12. The Psychology of Color in Marketing and Branding. www.helpscout.net. [Online] August 6, 2013. [Cited: March 4, 2014.] https://www.helpscout.net/blog/psychology-of-color/.

13. The Interactive Effects of Colors and Products on Perceptions of Brand Logo Appropriateness. Bottomley, P.A. and Doyle, J.R. 1: 63-83, s.l. : Marketing Theory, 2006, Vol. 6.

14. Are You Selling the Right Color? A Cross-Cultural Review of Color as a Marketing Cue. Aslam, Mubeen M. Cyprus, University of Wollongong : InterCollege, Marketing Department, School of Business Administration, 2005. UOW Library: research-pubs@uow.edu.au.

15. Ciotti, Gregory. www.kissmetrics.com. 7 Marketing

Lessons from Eye-Tracking Studies. [Online] 2013. [Cited: April 22, 2014.] http://blog.kissmetrics.com/eye-tracking-studies/.

16. Young, Scott. A Campaign for Improvement: Getting More From Print Advertising. [Online] Perception Research Services International, Inc, 2014. [Cited: April 22, 2014.] http://www.prsresearch.com/prs-insights/articel/a-campaign-for-improvement-getting-more-from-print-advertising.

17. Bindley, Katherine. Resume Design: Eye-Tracking Study Finds Job Seekers Have Six Seconds To Make An Impression Video. [Online] Huffington Post, May 9, 2012. [Cited: April 22, 2014.] http://www.huffingtonpost.com/2012/05/09/resume-design-eye-tracking-study-6-seconds.

18. Conducting Employment Interviews - Hiring How To. WSJ.com. [Online] The Wall Street Journal, 2009. [Cited: October 19, 2014.] http://guides.wsj/management.

19. Doyle, Alison. Behavioral Interviews (How to Prepare and Questions). Job Search. [Online] [Cited: October 28, 2014.] http://jobsearch.about.com.

About the Author

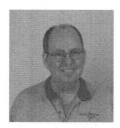

Dr. Steve Passmore graduated as a physical therapist in 1977 and has enjoyed a unique career. He has worked in hospitals, outpatient clinics, home health, rehab contract companies, and for the past 14 years in his own consulting company. His clinical years included experience in Management, Consultant for Advertising / Special Projects, Chief Operating Officer, Consultant for Recruiting, Clinical Vice President, and various other levels. His current company (Healthy Recruiting Tools) specializes in healthcare recruiting & software; plus a separate division (Focused Mailing Services) for direct mail advertising.

Healthy Recruiting Tools *– est. 2002 – Offering Professional Grade Recruiting Tools specifically designed for Management & Recruiters hiring Therapists, Nurses, and other Allied Health Professionals. Our "Tools" include: Direct Mail, Card Design, Enhanced Lists (we have the largest database of therapists in the industry), Software, Cold Calling (Hourly Cold Calls w/ $0 Placement Fees), & Recruiting In-Services.* www.RecruitingTherapy.com

Also, check out our direct mail company for commercial advertising. www.FocusedMailing.com

Would you like to utilize our Recruiting Tools?

Healthy Recruiting Tools
President: Dr. Steve Passmore
Contact: spass@HealthyRecruiting.com
Phone: (888) 993-9675
Products Include

- Hourly Cold Calling
  - Zero placement fees
  - We work on an hourly basis for a company to give you professional calling services as needed
  - NO RoBo-Calls
- List Enhancement
  - For larger companies with recruiting teams, we use our methods to obtain and enhance licensure lists. We simply create the best lists in the industry and have names the others miss. (Nurses / Therapists / Many other healthcare fields). Buy your lists through us and receive fresh data, we are the broker.
- We attach phone numbers to lists
- Recruiting software designed for healthcare
- Personal Recruiting Page (PRP)
  - Web page that specifically promotes your opening
- Direct mail services
  - Discount mail rates and materials
    - Oversize cards
    - Letters and inserts
    - Includes typical custom design or we can work with your current design
  - Best lists in the industry (Therapist, Nurse, and more)
  - Larger companies join our list-mail discount program
- Also providing traditional direct mail for advertising
- In-service training available to companies or state meetings

Contact us... to discuss affordable and effective options.

Made in the USA
Middletown, DE
03 April 2016